The Shades of Grief and The Uniqueness of You

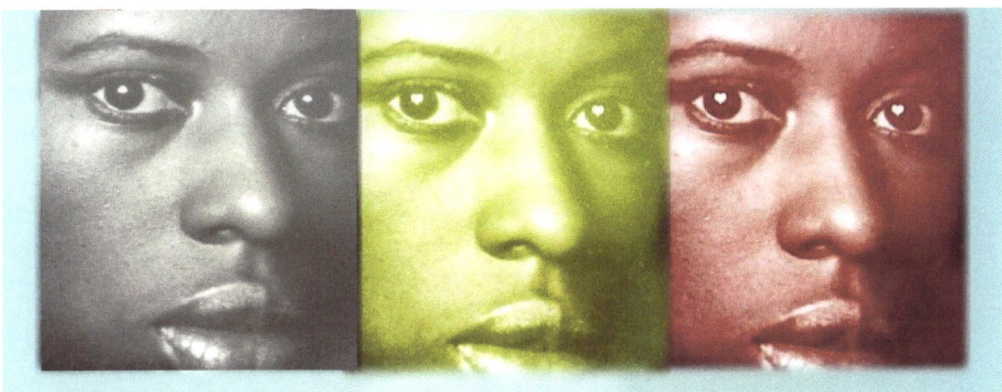

How to manage Grief by Finding Your Uniqueness Using Imagination, Creativity, Spirituality and the Power of Story

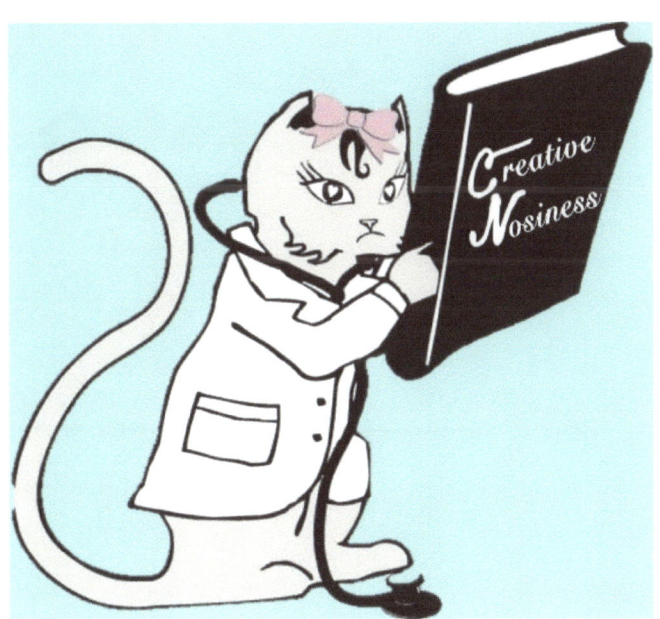

The Shades of Grief and the Uniqueness of You

All Rights Reserved

Copyright © 2018 by Dr. Audrey Pullman

All rights reserved. No part of this book may be used or reproduced by any means, graphic, electronic, or mechanical, including photocopying, recording, taping or by any information storage retrieval system without the written permission of the publisher except in the case of brief quotations embodied in critical articles and reviews.

- ISBN-13: 978-1726498333
- ISBN-10: 1726498336

- Published by: The Center for Writing Excellence, a Small Press
- Printed in the United States of America
- Date: September 2018

Other books and CDs by Dr. Audrey Pullman

For information, please contact Dr. Pullman at AudreyPullman@gmail.com

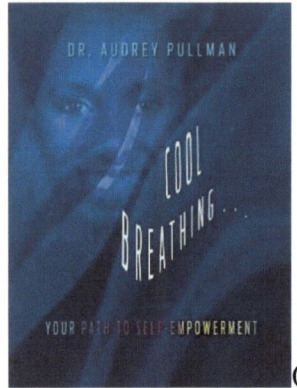
Cool Breathing, Your Path to Self-Empowerment

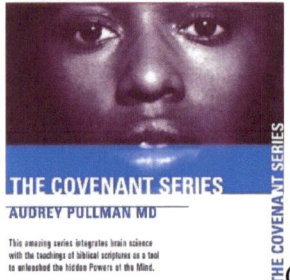
Covenant Series CD

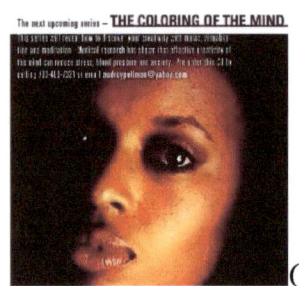
Coloring of the Mind CD

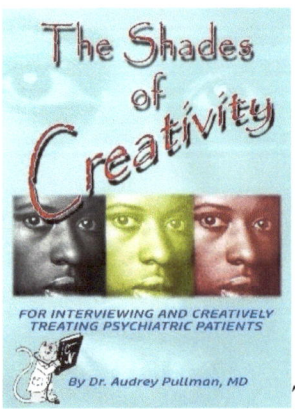
The Shades of Creativity

Table of Contents

The Uniqueness of You 1
Grief: No Pills Required!!! 3
What Causes Depression? 5
What is the Difference Between Grief and Depression? 7
Should Grief be Treated with Psychiatric Medications? 8
    Dr. Sidney Zisook 8
    Natural Emotions 10
Audrey Pullman's Story of Pain and Heartbreak 15
The OZ Principle 17
    Key Points 17
John W. James 19
Ms. Lois Hall 20
The Grief Recovery Method Principles 23
    The Grief Recovery Support Group 23
    Face the Pain 23
Grief and the Puerto Rico Connection 25
Grief and Creativity 29
The Power of Story 32
The Power of Story Exercises 37
    The Us Story 37
    You as The Story Teller and Director 37
        The Power of Story 1 - Vision 37
        The Power of Story 2 – Auditory 39
        The Power of Story 3 – Kinesthetic 41
The Shaman and I 45
Motivating Yourself 47
    Imagination 47

The Imagination Exercise – The Hot Air Balloon	48
Visualization = Goal Setting	52
The Waterfall Exercise	52
Meditation = The Language of Love, Peace, and Mind Power	53
A Ball of Confusion State of Mind	54
Tenacity and Resolve	**Error! Bookmark not defined.**
Cool Breathing	57
Eight Effective Breathing Techniques	60
Movement	69
Movement and Breathing Techniques	70
Cognitive Process	71
Dance and Brain	72
The Telomere Effect	75
What Methods Could Increase Telomeres? Meditation Yoga	76
Method 1 - The Mantra	77
The Meditation Yoga Research	77
Practice	78
The Power is in the Hands	78
Method 2 – Enhancing Telomerase	80
Love and Intimacy	80
Method 3 – Friendship and Social Activities	81
Method 4 – Nature and You	83
Reflection	86
The Umbrella Story	86
Your World is Upside Down	87
Your World is Cloudy	87
Your World is Full of Sunshine	88
A Reflection of a Balanced Life	88

- A World of Peace, Happiness and Joy 88
- Spirituality and the Grief Connection 89
  - The Grief Connection 89
- Psalms 23 – The Word 95
- A Letter to The American Psychiatry Association 99
- The Shades of Black 101
  - Revealing the Secrets of the Brain 101
  - The Mental Illness Stigma (*Shades of Black*) 101
- The Coloring of the Mind 105
  - The Dialogue 106
- Reference List 107
- Conclusion – a new life path 107

The Uniqueness of You

There is a surplus of grief books on the market that describe how individuals should recover from grief. Most authors' definition of grief describes a one-size-fits-all. Since we live in a multi-cultural society with various personalities, it's difficult to tell people how to grieve. This book is to provide you with creative tools to discover your uniqueness and manage your own grief – Creatively.

This book is unique because you will have to work toward unleashing your imagination and creativity while you grieve. This is a self-pace book and the reader will decide the best time, place and method of creative treatments to facilitate the grieving process. My motto for the grieving process is to do what you need to do and feel what you need to feel to heal.

Many grief writers do agree that Grief is an emotional heartbreak. This book will allow you the reader to determine which tools to use to mend your broken heart.

The goal is to provide you with a sense of creative self-empowerment. Each one of us have our own creative artistic fingerprint which is derived from our DNA and uniqueness on how we see the world.

Are you one of a kind? Then you must have unique quality that makes you stand out from all of the rest. This book will help you discover your uniqueness even in the darkest periods of your life.

Grief: No Pills Required!!!

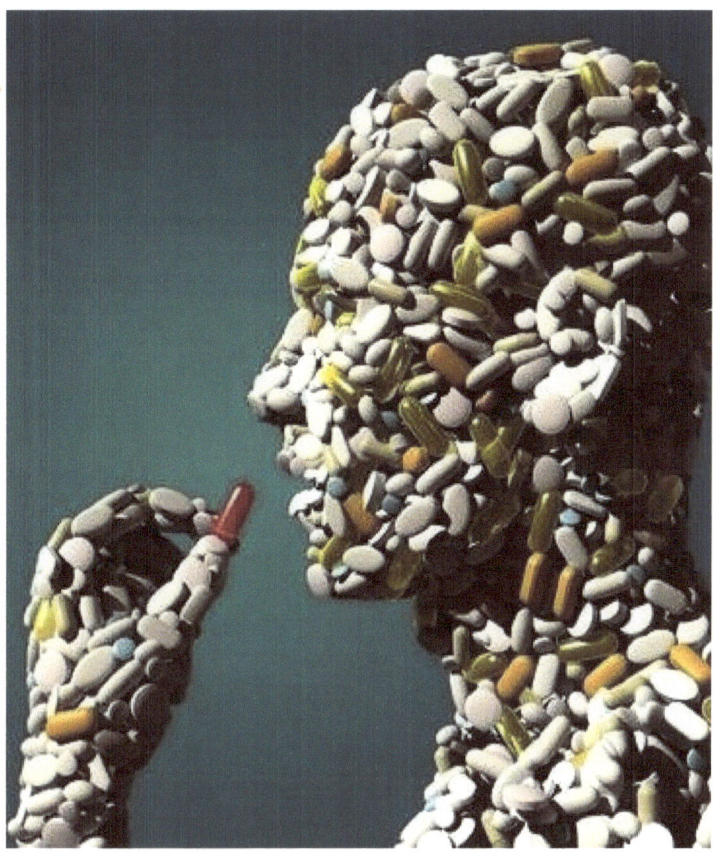

As a trained psychiatrist, I know the signs and symptoms of Grief. The American Psychiatry Association (APA) defines prolonged bereavement/ Grief Reaction, IC9 code – V6280 as the following:

Depression Is Different from Sadness or Grief/Bereavement

The death of a loved one, loss of a job or the ending of a relationship are difficult experiences for a person to endure. It is normal for feelings of sadness or grief to develop in response to such situations. Those experiencing loss often might describe themselves as being "depressed."

But being sad is not the same as having depression. The grieving process is natural and unique to everyone and shares some of the same features of depression. Both grief and depression may involve intense sadness and withdrawal from usual activities. They are also different in important ways:

- In grief, painful feelings come in waves, often intermixed with positive memories of the deceased. In major depression, mood and/or interest (pleasure) are decreased for most of two weeks.
- In grief, self-esteem is usually maintained. In major depression, feelings of worthlessness and self-loathing are common.
- For some people, the death of a loved one can bring on major depression. Losing a job or being a victim of a physical assault or a major disaster can lead to depression for some people. When grief and depression co-exist, the grief is more severe and lasts longer than grief without depression. Despite some overlap between grief and depression, they are different. Distinguishing between them can help people get the help, support or treatment they need.

In medical school I learned the following acronym for clinical depression: **SIG E CAPS**

Sleep   (Decreased)

Interest   (Decreased)

Guilt   (Feelings of Guilt)

Energy   (Decreased Energy)

Concentration   (Decreased

Appetite   (Decreased)

Psychomotor retardation or slow movement

Suicide ideation

Clinical depression can range from mild, moderate or to severe. Grief has an impact on the heart and depression on the brain. Science tracks the seat of our emotions to the brain. It's often said that depression results from a chemical imbalance. However, clinical depression is more complicated than that. Researchers believe that certain areas of the brain help regulate mood – more important than levels of specific brain chemicals-nerve cell connections, nerve cell growth, and the functioning of nerve circuits have a major impact on depression. Therefore, there are many possible causes of depression, including faulty mood regulation by the brain, genetic vulnerability, stressful life events, medications, and medical problems.

What Causes Depression?

Cause #1 for Depression

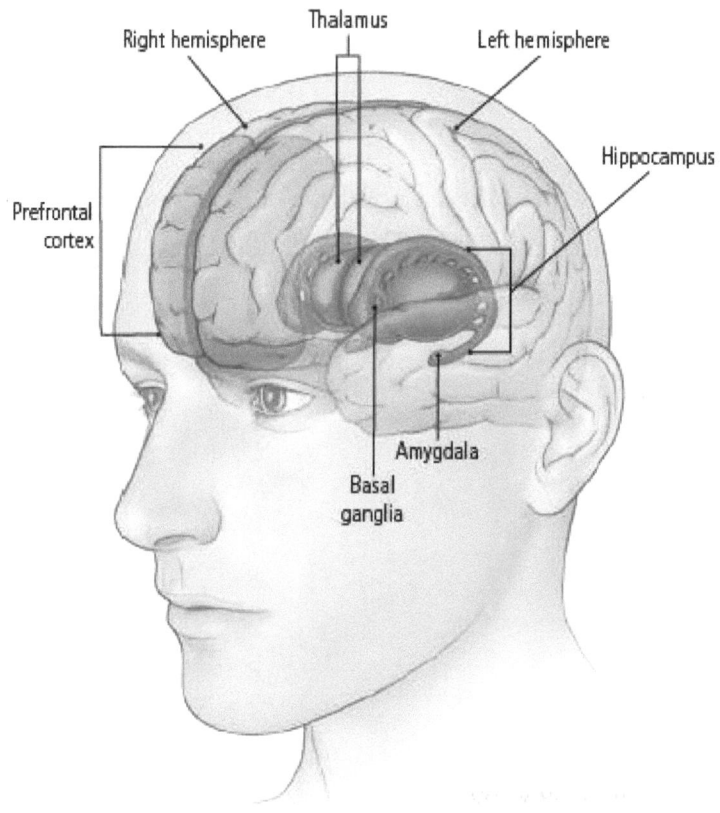

The regions shown here are mirrored in both hemispheres of the brain. Also, these structures are interlocking; the illustration suggests location and relative region but not precise location.

Amygdala: The amygdala is part of the limbic system, a group of structures deep in the brain that's associated with emotions such as anger, pleasure, sorrow, fear, and sexual arousal. The amygdala is activated when a person recalls emotionally charged memories, such as a frightening situation. Activity in the amygdala is higher when a person is sad or clinically depressed. This increased activity continues even after recovery from depression.

Thalamus: The thalamus receives most sensory information and relays it to the appropriate part of the cerebral cortex, which directs high-level functions such as speech, behavioral reactions, movement, thinking, and learning. Some research suggests that bipolar disorder may result from problems in the thalamus, which helps link sensory input to pleasant and unpleasant feelings.

Hippocampus: The hippocampus is part of the limbic system and has a central role in processing long-term memory and recollection. Interplay between the hippocampus and the amygdala might account for the adage "once bitten, twice shy." It is this part of the brain that registers fear when you are confronted by a barking, aggressive dog, and the memory of such an experience may make you wary of dogs you come across later in life. The hippocampus is smaller in some depressed people, and research suggests that ongoing exposure to stress hormone impairs the growth of nerve cells in this part of the brain.

Cause #2 for Depression

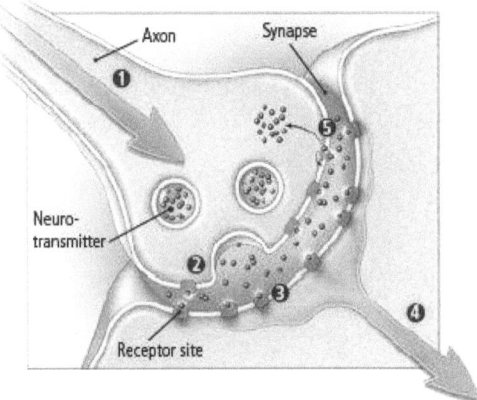

1. An electrical signal travels down the axon.
2. Chemical neurotransmitter molecules are released.
3. The neurotransmitter molecules bind to receptor sites.
4. The signal is picked up by the second neuron and is either passed along or halted.

The signal passed along the second neuron causing a reuptake, the process by which the cell that released the neurotransmitter takes back some of the remaining molecules. However, when this reuptake is affected and there is a depletion in neurotransmitters due to faulty mood regulation by the brain, genetic vulnerability, stressful life events, medications, and medical problems; this could lead to the onset of major depression.

What is the Difference Between Grief and Depression?

In 2011 I filed a discrimination lawsuit and I won my case in September 2017. During those six horrible years I never felt suicidal, but I did exhibit the following symptoms of Grief:

1. Sadness, despair, mourning
2. Fatigue or low energy
3. Tears
4. Loss of appetite
5. Poor sleep
6. Poor concentration
7. Happy and sad memories
8. Mild feelings of guilt

Grief has several symptoms in common with major depressive disorder, including intense sadness, insomnia, poor appetite and weight loss. In fact, the symptoms of grief and depression can appear remarkable similar.

Getting the correct diagnosis is essential for appropriate treatment, so a comprehensive medical and psychological exam is often done.

With grief it is normal to experience sadness and cry. It is normal to experience changes in sleep patterns, energy levels and appetite. It is normal to have difficulty concentrating and to have moments of anger, loneliness, and more. The difference, with grief, is that these feelings of sadness usually begin to debate over time. However, clues that you may be suffering with major depressive disorder include:

9. Feelings of guilt not related to the loved one's death.
10. Thoughts of suicide-although in grief there can be thoughts of "joining" the deceased.
11. Morbid preoccupation with worthlessness (grief does not usually erode self-confidence).
12. Sluggishness or hesitant and confused speech.
13. Prolonged and Marked difficulty in carrying out the activities of day-to-day living.
14. Hallucinations and delusions.

Should Grief be Treated with Psychiatric Medications?

"NO"! While grief can be extremely painful, there is generally no medical indication to treat it. There are exception, if their secondary causes for grief-related symptoms, such as, anxiety or sleep disturbances.

Grieving is a highly individual process for each person and determining when normal grief becomes complicated grief can be difficult. There's currently no consensus among mental health experts about how much time must pass before complicated grief can be diagnosed.

Complicated grief may be considered when the intensity of grief has not decreased in the months after your loved one's death. Some mental health professionals diagnose complicated grief when grieving continues to be intense, persistent and debilitating beyond 12 months

Prior to prescribing any medications for complicated grief the key is to consider other treatment modalities such as, psychotherapy. This treatment can be effective when done individually or in a group format.

Grievers will also benefit from grief support groups and 1:1 sessions with a grief specialist. I recommend exploring the Grief Recovery Method program. This is an action program that will allow you to explore your grief through writing letters, a timeline graph, and other modalities to face your pain. The staff are professional people who will show you compassion and understanding toward finding your uniqueness on how to cope with fear, anxiety and unlock the potential of your life.

Dr. Sidney Zisook

The American Psychiatric Association and the new language for Grief–DSM-5

Dr. Sidney Zisook is a renowned Psychiatrist with a specialty in Grief. He was my former Psychiatry Director when I did my internship at The University of San Diego School of Medicine (UCSD).

He is a Distinguished Professor of Psychiatry at UCSD. He served as an advisor to the DSM-5's Mood Disorder Work Group. Dr. Zisook's does research on mood as both a primary and secondary manifestation/disorder. Much of his research has been focused on the natural history, differentiation from depression and treatment of grief and bereavement.

I had the opportunity to meet with Dr. Zisook several years ago at his UCSD office to discuss my idea on how to integrate creative ideas to treat patients into the standard medical school curriculum. He would provide me the opportunity to speak with his third and fourth year psychiatry residents.

During our conversation he discussed being on the work group that changed some of the ways that grief and clinical depression were described and differentiated in the new diagnostic and Statistical Manual of Mental Disorders, typically referred to as DSM-5. Several of his colleagues was upset with the elimination of, "bereavement exclusion." The "exclusion" essentially detailed a two-month period of "normal grief" that people would experience after the loss of a loved one. During this period, it was all but forbidden to diagnose a patient with major depression-even if the individual had all the symptoms. Dr. Zisook felt that the definition of bereavement had evolved, and this restriction was based on the best science from the mid-1980s, the last time DSM was fully revised, but the science of bereavement and major depressive disorder has changed.

Dr. Zisook work group found the exclusion was too limiting; normal grief often lasts much longer than two months, and a small subset of patients can have major depression triggered or exacerbated by a loved one's death, just as they can from all kinds of loses and traumas. Per Dr. Zisook, *February 25, 2013, Guest Blog, "Getting Past the Grief over Grief,* "critics have convinced a lot of people that the work group goal was to diagnose every grieving person with major depressive disorder."

Dr. Zisook explained to his colleagues who disagreed with these changes that, "dropping the exclusion does not re-label grief as major depression, nor does it medicalize grief." "That is not to suggest grief is not "depressing." For many people, grief is very depressing, but those emotions are not the same as having a major depressive disorder, a serious clinical condition that certainly is not part of a normal grief."

Why did the work group change the grief language in DSM-5? Read more at: https://blogs.scientificamerican.com/guest-blog/getting-past-the-grief-over-grief

Dr. Zisook states, "that his work group changed the grief language in DSM-5 to make sure clinicians and patients understand that major depression can occur in someone who is bereaved, just as it can occur in someone who is going through a divorce, facing a sudden disability or terminal illness, or struggling with serious financial troubles."

"There are no known clinically meaningful differences in the severity, course or treatment response of major depressive episodes that occur after the death of a loved one compared to those occurring in any other context."

Finally, Dr. Zisook states, "According to the best research available, any very stressful life event can trigger a major depressive episode in a vulnerable person; regardless of the context in which it occurs, prompt recognition and appropriate treatment can be life-promoting and even life-saving."

Additional article on the DSM-V bereavement exclusion:

https://www.ncbi.nlm.nih.gov/pmc/articles/pmc2922362, *The Bereavement exclusion for the diagnosis of major depression:* Kristy Lamb, MD, Ronald Pies, MD and Sidney Zisook, MD

Natural Emotions

Naturally occurring is an authentic and powerful emotion. A lot of people don't know how to tap into these emotions to provide them with support and stability. For example, Love is a natural emotion-it evokes a certain response or feeling when you meet the person you love. We didn't have to learn or rehearse how to respond to love because our human to human emotions unleashes certain hormones that transmit to our neurons and releases "a feel good" response to this intense feeling of affection. When this positive feeling is taken away from us through an emotional heartbreak we become imbalanced and unhappy due to this negative emotion transformation that takes over our mind, body and spirit.

This book will guide you on how to explore grief creatively to uncover your creative fingerprint. Once this happens it can lead you to creative self-empowerment which will allow you to become more confident in your decision making. This will bring an emotional balance on how to manage your feelings both in the good and bad times. As humans we have many emotions to display our personality, character and state of mind.

Mr. Jordan Gray (https:/www.jordangrayconsulting.com) states in his article, *"What Our Emotions Are Trying to Tell Us."* Mr. Jordan list and explain five core emotions from this article: Happiness, Sadness, Sexual, Anger and Fear.

1. Happiness

This is our default emotional reality when our basic human needs are being met.

We feel happy when we feel safe, connected, and loved.

On one end of the spectrum of arousal happy can feel like calm, relaxed contentment, and the other side of the spectrum it can register as joy, bliss, ecstasy, or the feeling of being in love.

Our bodies often feel expanded, warm, flowing, and relaxed when we are happy.

2. Sadness

Sadness flows through our bodies when we are experiencing some form of loss in our lives. Whether that loss is around something as contextually insignificant as dropping our ice cream cone on the ground, or as devastating as the end of a relationship or losing a job or a loved one that we adored.

People go to great lengths to avoid allowing themselves to feel sadness. But I like to think of sadness as a kind of honoring process. We honor how much something meant to us when we let the ripples of sadness flow through our body... whether in a temporary pouting kind of way, or in a take several days or weeks to full-out sob when we experience a more significant loss in our lives.

And it's true... you can feel it to heal it. If you let yourself lean into your emotional processing of sadness, it will one day flow through you and you can heal your way to the bottom of it. Allowing yourself to fully experience sadness will only make you a stronger and more resilient person.

Physical symptoms of sadness often include a feeling of heaviness in your chest, tension around your jaw and throat muscles, and tears in your eyes.

3. Sexual

Out of the five emotions on this list, I would say that this one is the most often neglected in other people's lists (because you could argue that it stems from happiness, but I feel like it's different enough and neglected enough in our culture that I'm going to include it... plus it's my list so I'll do what I want).

Sexual arousal is experienced differently from person to person, but common physical experiences often feel like some combination of a feeling of heat in the chest and groin area, visible redness or flushing of the face and upper chest, a slowing down of the pacing of your breathing, and a spreading feeling of the arousal eventually making its way through your entire body.

Our sexual desire is one of the strongest driving forces in our entire lives (after all, it *is* responsible for our species thriving). When you learn how to harness your sexual energy you can feel unstoppable. Our sexual energy can be transmuted into creative energy, and it is a force unlike any other.

It's also important to remember that your sexual energy (just like every emotion that you experience) is created by you and lives only in your body. So even though it's easy to think, "I saw that attractive person and they turned me on", in reality, you turned yourself on. Just like people don't "make" you sad, angry, or happy, we have to learn to take personal responsibility for our own emotions. This is often the case with our sexual feelings even more than the others.

4. Anger

Mr. Jordan states, "one of the coolest things that I ever learned when studying childhood development (whether this is true or not I don't really care, I just like the idea of it) is that we can't learn to crawl until we learn the emotion of anger (or the secondary emotion in this particular example would be frustration). We can't crawl because we must be angry enough about our current situation of not being able to move ourselves around. We want to be mobile, and we resent the limitation of being stationary. Enter anger… and then the learning moment follows."

Anger is the feeling that we are either being blocked in some way (there is an obstacle between us and our desired outcome) or that we are getting something that we don't want. An example of the former would be a sumo wrestler attempting to push his opponent out of the ring, and an example of the latter would be someone trying to take credit for work that we did in a job that we held close to our sense of identity. The former is proactive, the latter is reactive.

When you're angry your muscles tighten up (jaw tensing, fists clenched, major muscle groups experiencing strain, etc.) and you feel like energy is trying to force its way out of your body. Whether that registers as pushing against something or someone, stomping our feet on the ground, or growing/making noises, anger causes us to act.

5. Fear

Fear is meant to keep us safe. But sometimes it overstays its welcome and it keeps us too safe (for example, fear of what other people will think of you could keep you from pursuing your dream career).

On the low end of the spectrum, you might experience fear as nerves… nerves before a first date, or before doing some public speaking for example.

We've all heard about some version of the fight or flight, or fight-flight-freeze response. The fight or flight response kicks in at a higher end of the spectrum when we perceive a threat that we believe could do actual damage to us (physically or emotionally).

But the important thing to recognize with our evolving minds is that we experience fear even when it doesn't serve us. We do this because we experience fear in response to the *perception* of a threat, not exclusively to actual threats. What does that mean? It means we feel fear even when we imagine or invent something to be afraid of, not just when there is a clear and certain threat to our well-being.

How do you overcome fear and start feeling better? How can you survive?

You may also not want to feel better. The thought of feeling better may feel disrespectful -- like trying to "let go" before you're ready. That's okay. Grief is not some sort of awkward, embarrassing "condition" that should be "gotten over" or "healed" as soon as possible.

Grief is our final expression of love, the last gift we have to offer. It isn't to be rushed. Our grief is a unique, yet universal, experience of a human being capable of loving. The more intense the feelings, the deeper the witness to the intensity of love shared.

If we cannot manage our emotions during these difficult times we could do things that make it worse. Such as turning to drugs, alcohol or other self-destructive behaviors to cope with our loss. It is more helpful to stay connected with our support system (e.g. family, friends and spiritual advisors) who can support and comfort us while we are dealing with a heartbreak. As much as you might want to isolate yourself it is usually very helpful to try to keep up with your daily routine.

If you're grieving over a long period of time and things appear to be getting worse this may indicate that you're having trouble handling the grief on your own. This is when it might be helpful to reach out to get professional help. I recommend contacting the below references to help you with managing your emotions at your time of grief.

References:

https://www.griefrecoverymethod.com/

https://www.audreygriefexpressionist.com

Audrey Pullman's Story of Pain and Heartbreak

As a Psychiatrist, I had extensive training in mental illness and the neuropathology of the human mind. I was well equipped to understand when my patients were experiencing grief. As human beings, we all have a loss in our life through a death of a loved one, a broken heart or a job loss. There was always a void in my heart with a death of a loved one. However, even though I would miss their presence, I would move on cultivating their memories.

As a disaster physician, I work with individuals who were affected by manmade and natural disasters (e.g. hurricanes, earthquakes & fire). In 2005, I was deployed to assist disaster survivors who was affected by Hurricane Katrina. Due to my disaster-related work performance I was recommended to work with a presidential appointee to open a new disability office. The office had no staff, and temporary workers were hired to ensure the success of this new office.

The five staff members worked long hours and we were proud of our successes and commitment to this new office. The disability director received funding to hire people to staff this new office. She offered me a position but said I had to compete and if I make the certification list which mean I was qualified for the job she could hired me directly. During my time in the office I served in many leadership roles and worked on a diversity of projects, committees, and even published a paper.

I had a lot to offer in the position and I, along with my co-workers, developed the positions in the office at headquarters. In all honesty, this seemed to be a rare situation where there was a good match and an opportune time for both the new office and the staff members, who in a sense pioneered the position. It just seemed that the time was right, and I was more than qualified for the position, but I didn't get it! I was very upset. I was hurt, devastated, and inconsolable. I shook, I couldn't catch my breath, and I sobbed uncontrollably. As I reflected on this time, I wonder why I acted so emotional for a job loss; no one died! However, I was part of a team that developed this new office for 12 months, and it's rare when my interest, background, determination, and on-the-job experience truly match the advertised position. I was experiencing a broken heart!

From 2011 to 2017, I had been more angry, bitter and frustrated than I have ever been. These feelings of sadness took over and dominated my life. I can truthfully say that I found myself in more emotional turmoil from 2011 to the present than I have ever experienced in any other time in my life. Emotional distress, pain and suffering, embarrassment, inconvenience, loss of enjoyment of life -- I had been deeply harmed in all these categories from 2011 to the present. These had been bitter, joyless years.

Beginning in 2016 I began to reclaim control of my life, but I still wasn't over it. My recovery was very slow, and uneven. The sadness, anger, and frustration were just below the surface, and many times a thought or memory will remind me all over again what happened to me in 2011. That is when all those miserable feelings flood back over me again. I had faith that recovery would occur for me, but my wounds were not healed yet, but I knew that I had to get off of this rollercoaster of not moving forward.

My life was in a pause phase of sadness and I was feeling sorry for myself daily. One evening I was watching the Wizard of Oz on television. This movie motivated me to do something with my life. I began with something simple. I asked myself, "What is the definition of grief?" Now I had learned about grief in medical school, but my training was incomplete. I also had my own business, *Audrey's Grief Expressionist, LLC* but I still didn't have a complete understanding of the definition of grief. I googled grief and I liked the definition from the Grief Recovery Method Institute. There definition was simple, "Grief is a Heartbreak." I went on the Grief Recovery website and read the Founder, John W. James biography and I was very impressed with his perseverance and motivation to solve problems for himself and grievers who didn't have anywhere to go find help.

Therefore, I began to move forward with my life from the Oz Principle motto: It was time to stop having a pity party and take control of my life. I embarked on a journey that would change my life - learning about the Grief Recovery Method Program.

The OZ Principle

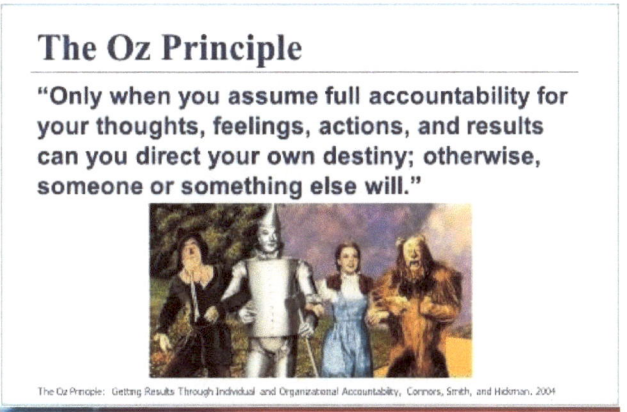

Key Points

In the Wizard of Oz, the 1939 American musical fantasy film produced by Metro-Goldwyn-Mayer, is the most well-known and commercially successful adaptation based on the 1900 novel, "The Wonderful Wizard of Oz," by L. Frank Baum. The film was nominated for Best Picture but lost to another picture you may have heard of entitled, "Gone with the Wind." Contrary to popular belief, the movie was not the first color film; there were others before The Wizard of Oz.

The Oz principle and like Dorothy and the gang in The Wizard of Oz, most people have the tools to succeed, but when things go wrong they blame circumstance or others instead of looking within for the true cause of unsatisfactory results. Once individuals learn to accept responsibility, they can use the Oz Principle to become better leaders.

Lion - if I only had courage

Tin Man - if I only had a heart

Scarecrow - if I only had a brain

They all blamed their inabilities on something that they perceived was lacking in themselves. They all thought they needed to get to OZ and the wizard, so he could give them what they were lacking. When they got to OZ they discovered that the wizard was a fake. They had in them all the time the traits that they thought they were lacking.

Control your own destiny by taking responsibility of your thoughts, feelings, actions and results. This includes learning how to manage life's many challenges and heartbreaks. Like most people after a loss, they need comfort and not treatment. I would also add that grievers need the courage to face their pain, feel comfortable displaying their natural emotions but like in the Oz principle use their heart and brain to take control over their emotional heartbreak.

My personal heartbreak was a six-year journey. I had medical colleagues who said I was grieving too long and I maybe suffering from depression. I reminded them that grieving is a personal and highly individual experience. How I grieve is component of my DNA, personality, coping style, life experience, faith and the nature of the loss. My grieving process took a long time. Some start to feel better in weeks or months. For others, the grieving process is measured in years.

I had a great support system with family and friends. As the years went by there was a slow easing of my pain. There were times when I had relapses when I was reminded of the pain. Perhaps my most vital steps in coping were integrating creativity during my prolonged grieving period. As a former actress and model, I would act out my pain. Creativity allowed me to feel free and do whatever it took to get unstuck. Such as writing down my feelings, crying my heart out, screaming my anger to the skies, or pounding out my guilt on the floor. Far from being childish, these actions let me get my feelings into the open. There I could look at them and begin to understand them, which was a healthy start on releasing them on my journey of healing. Know that it is your right to be upset.

During the six years of loss I experienced a lot of anger. When this emotion would escalate it began to affect my mental clarity. This is the time I sought spiritual guidance from my mother, Minister Joann Pullman Silas. She informed me that focusing anger on a target of blame is a distraction. Also, if I focus on only one strong emotion at a time, it would sap my energy and I would have little time to feel and face my pain. Mom said acknowledging my pain is an essential part of the grieving process, so while the distraction of anger may temporarily seem to ease my feelings, in the long run, it only serves to prolong an already unbearable situation.

John W. James

The Grief Recovery Method Program Founder: John W. James

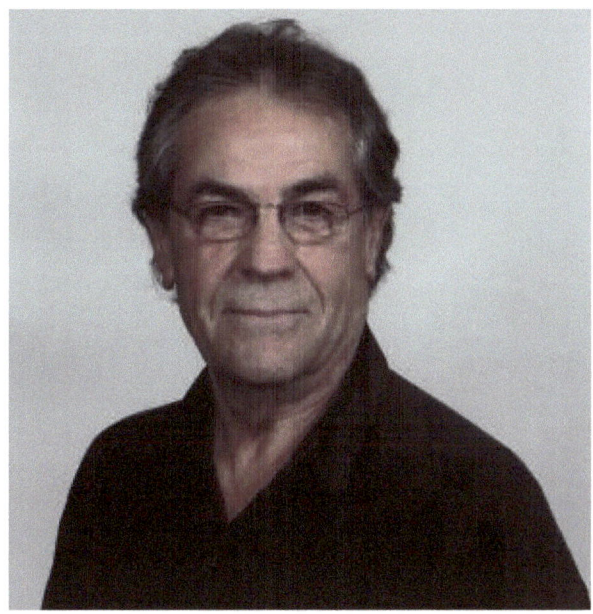

Biography and picture taken from **WWW.GRIEF**recoverymethod.com

John W. James was born in Danville, Illinois. He was thrust unwillingly into the arena of grief and recovery when his three-day-old son died in 1977. **John W. James** founded the Grief Recovery Institute forty years ago as a solution when he couldn't find the resources he needed to deal with his own overwhelming grief at the death of his infant son. Since then the institute has expanded to include sister organizations in Canada, England, Sweden and Mexico. Mr. James states, "Our mission is to deliver grief recovery assistance to the largest number of people in the shortest amount of time." John is internationally recognized as one of the foremost authorities on grief in the world today.

I embarked on finding a grief program that would require me to act in healing my broken heart due to race and gender discrimination. I discovered the Grief Recovery Method Support programs that have been developed and refined over the past 30 years, they teach you how to recover from loss. This intense action program is exactly what I needed to work toward my healing process.

Ms. Lois Hall

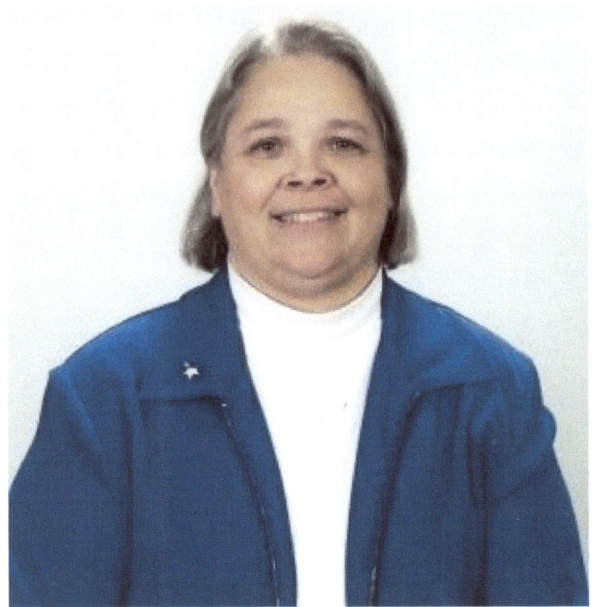

Since I am a Psychiatrist, I know many colleagues that could have easily provided psychotherapy for me with the standard approach of diagnosed and treat which only would have magnify my sense of failure and heartbreak. As a physician, I was trained in alternative medicine to treat the whole person, and I was looking for a program who would be my ally and understood that wellness is a very individual and personal issue. I found this ally in Ms. Lois Hall, who area of specialty is grief recovery. She has been facilitating community-based Grief Recovery Method Support Groups since 1998 and was invited to become a trainer for the Grief Recovery Institute in 2002.

The key component of this four-day group sessions is to focus on optimal well-being. Ms. Hall didn't focus on the diagnosis and treatment of illness; rather, the goal of helping me achieve the highest level of mental and physical health possible. It was a positive approach that implied self-motivation action. My group recovery sessions with Ms. Hall required me to investigate myself, to acknowledge my heartbreak but to build upon my inner strength to confront my fears and disappointments. I attended the four-day Group Recovery Method program from February 13 – 17, 2016.

Prior to attending the program, I spoke with a grief recovery representative and explained my reasons for wanting to attend this course which was due to the loss of a job promotion in 2011. This was a life changing event and caused me to have feelings of sadness, anxiety, loss of self-worth and appetite, as well as altered sleep patterns. I recommend anyone who wants to begin the process of healing from any emotionally or traumatic event to contact the Grief Recovery Method program.

The Grief Recovery Method Principles

What I liked about the Grief Recovery program is three-folded: First, I felt safe in the class environment. Secondly, upon my arrival I met the warmness and kindness of Ms. Hall that allowed me to feel free and not intimidated or overwhelmed about the process. Thirdly, this is an action-based program that you have to become an active partner in feeling better. Finally, at the closing of each class sessions we all would stand in a circle, placing one foot forward and hugging each other. For me, this triggered a powerful of emotion of support, love, connection and the oneness of emotional togetherness.

The Grief Recovery Support Group

The Grief Recovery process began each morning from 8:30am to 5:30pm. I was taught the following principles to facilitate my grief recovery healing:

- The Grief Recovery Method Principles, what is grief?
- What is incomplete loss and how to identify the loss?
- Concepts of Recovery and Homework assignments
- Practice Application Training
- How to heal a broken heart?
- Development of Completion Exercises

Initially discussing my loss was difficult and the resultant pain from that loss. However, receiving feedback, understanding and compassion from other people in the group was very effective. Also writing out a timeline of my loss and sending letters to some of the people who had been involved with me during that traumatic event, helped facilitate my grieving process.

Face the Pain

During this intensive four-day process at the Grief Recovery program I had to "Face the Pain" of my heartbreak; something I was resistant to do. I treated my pain privately and I had difficulty sharing my pain amongst strangers in a group setting. I had discussed my grief on a superficial level and I was very resistant to crying, seeking and accepting the group support.

The instructor, Ms. Lois Hall, was very caring and personable. My private exterior began to break when Ms. Hall introduced the team to the Loss History Graph Timeline. The Founder Mr. John James and his partner Mr. Russell Friedman developed this wonderful exercise. This timeline can be found in their book, *"The Grief Recovery Handbook, pages 87-90*. Per book authors, the primary purpose of this exercise is to create a detailed examination of the loss events in your life and to identify the patterns that have resulted from them. Some of these patterns are painful and some are not. I learned from this training how to be a good steward of my pain because it involves feeling alive again.

Face the Pain Examples:

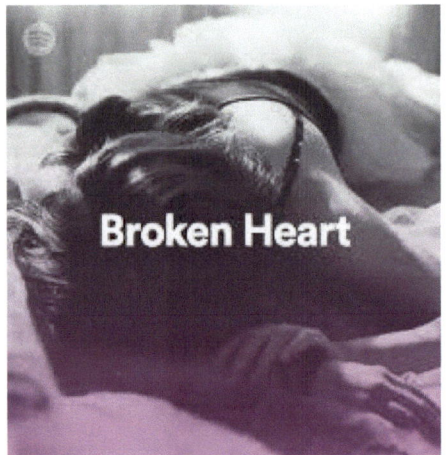

If your heart is heavy from a broken heart: Face the Pain!

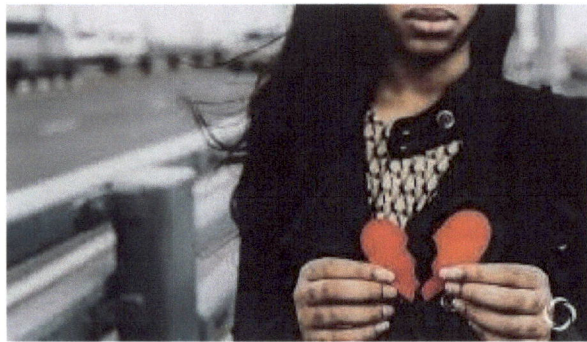

Grief and the Puerto Rico Connection

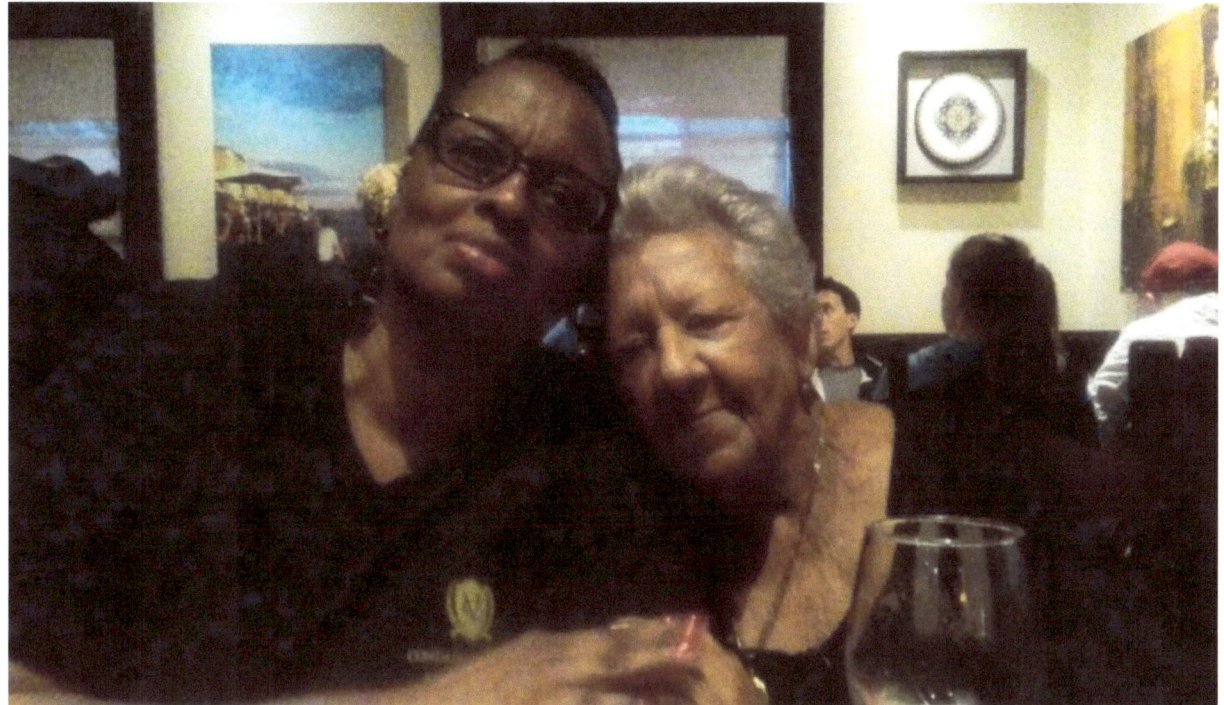

Dr. Audrey Pullman Graham and Mrs. Lu Lu Gonzales, a disaster survivor.

I have a 14 year history of disaster deployment work. I have done grief work in many disasters from hurricane Katrina to hurricane Maria. The mission is to help survivors recover from their grief and to provide disaster relief for some of their personal loses through local, state and federal assistance.

I was deployed to Puerto Rico on November 14, 2017 and didn't return home until July 3, 2018. Puerto Rico had been devastated by Hurricane Maria, a powerful Category 4 storm that also impacted several islands in the Caribbean. It was the strongest storm to make landfall in 85 years. The devastation to this beautiful island was unbelievable. It came ashore on September 20, 2017 with sustained winds of 155 mph, knocking out power to the entire island. Trees were uprooted, homes were destroyed, and there was also widespread flooding.

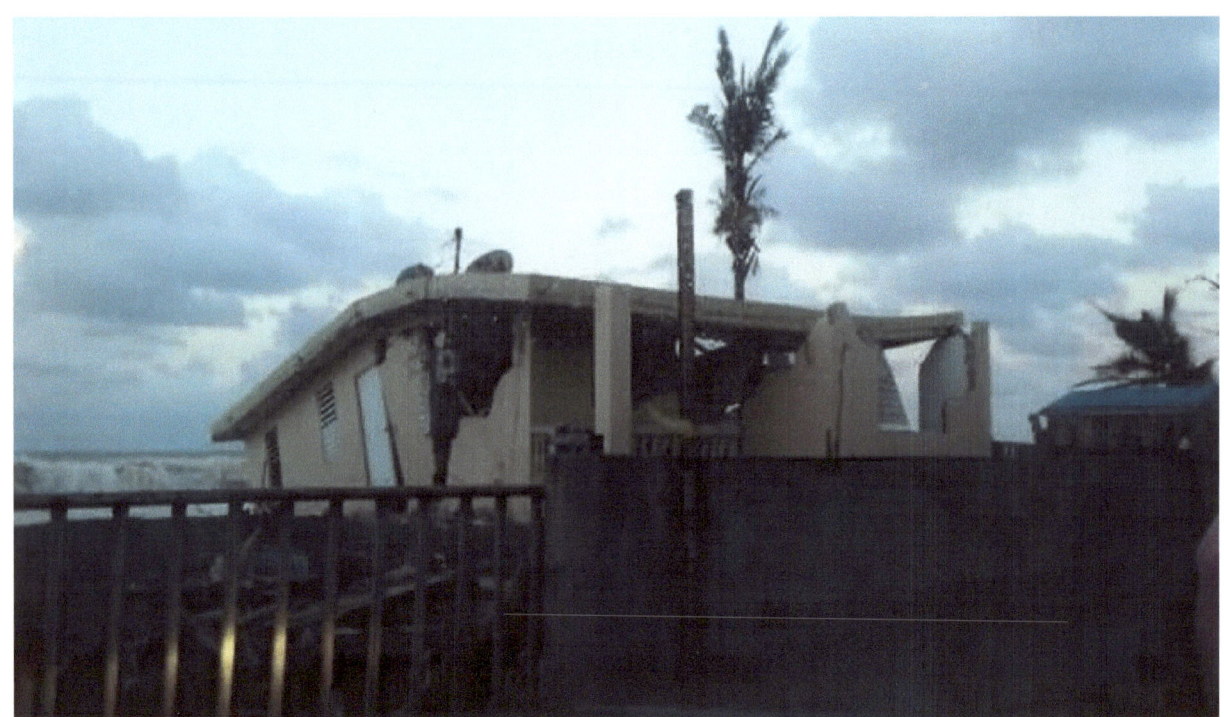

I have a special place in my heart for Puerto Rico because I completed my last few years of medical education at the Universidad Del Caribe School of Medicine. It was awesome that I could returned to help the islanders with their grief and to advise them how to get federal assistance. I was assigned to work as a disability supervisor in the rural areas of this island. Many people were still without utilities. The traffic lights were nonexistent. Cars were still underwater, and transportation was very limited.

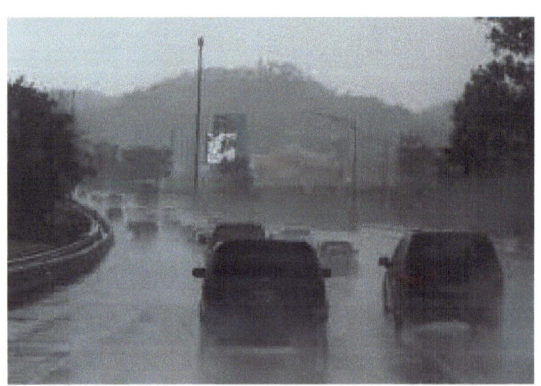

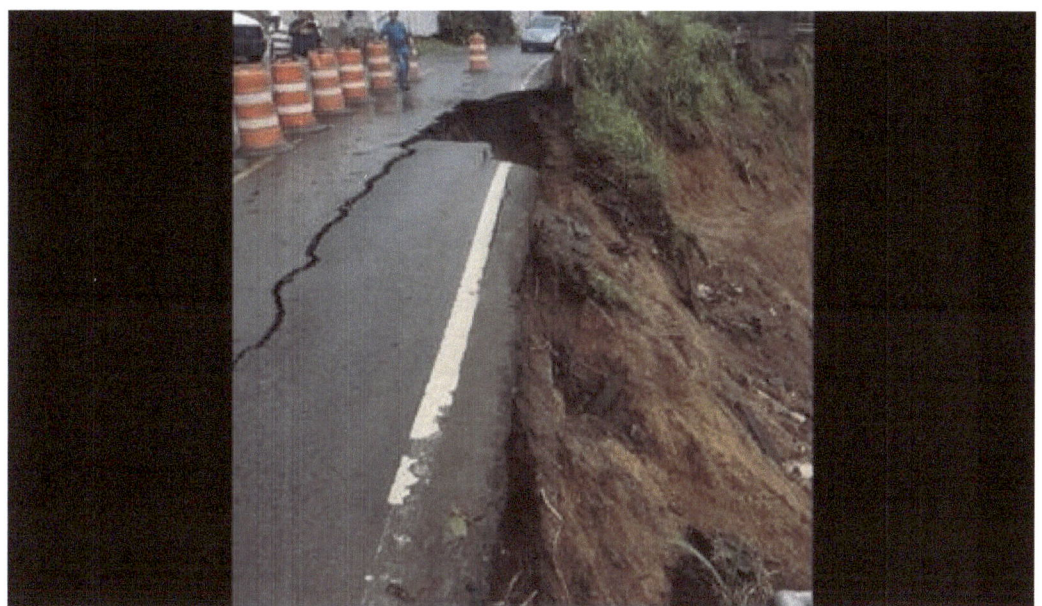

The Oracovis municipality in Puerto Rico is a mountainous area and the driving was very treacherous. I had a wonderful person, CJ who was an American Sign Language interpreter on my team. He drove me to areas that were very dangerous. CJ had no fear! Our goal was to help the survivors! There were teams of people in Puerto Rico who were non-volunteers and volunteers that came to the island to help. As we explored these areas we could see power lines scattered across the roads in Orocovis and saw numerous homes and personal property damages.

The islanders continue to be strong and strive toward overcoming such significant heartbreak and pain.

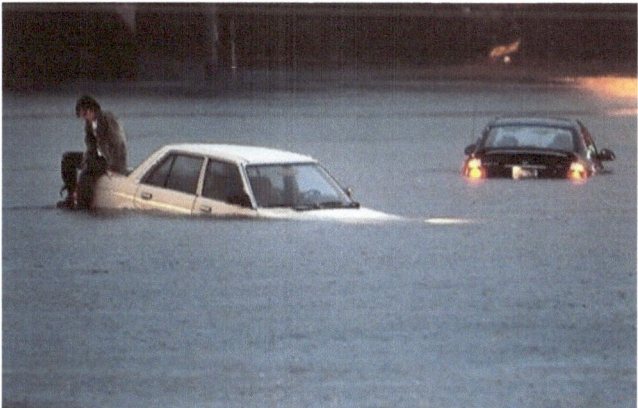

Grief and Creativity

Every human being will experience grief in their life time. Grief is a journey we all must endure after the loss of a loved one. Don't listen to professionals who tell you how long and how you should grieve. This is your own personal journey. Creativity allows you to express your grief in your own unique way. The best way to work through grief is to let it out. Cry, scream, and yell if you need to. These types of outlets provide a healthy emotional release and help clear out the cobwebs. Express your feelings through music, art, poetry, or journaling. Whether you express your grief with a safe person you trust or let it out in complete privacy, expressing your pain and feelings is the only true way to honor your grief and begin to work through it.

I currently work with medical students and physicians on how to handle the loss of their patients, and to take care of themselves after this loss. As physicians, we often develop close relationships with our patients, and may eventually lose one. Grief-related job stress may become job-related burnout, which can affect up to 50 percent of physicians treating terminally ill patients. It's important for physicians affected by the loss of a patient to find a healthy way to cope.

I've written two books on self-care using creativity for the physicians and their patients. My books focus on creative self-empowerment and how to manage grief in the best and worst of times. It's important to "Let emotions happen, it makes you human and empathetic. It takes time to get over a death, and it is okay to remember those that have died.

Make no mistake, establishing a creative practice takes effort, commitment, and discipline, just like many of the most worthwhile things in life. But it will reward you, again and again. Creativity can become a cornerstone of your life, as well as a pathway through grief, and a stimulant of huge growth.

Creativity shares a trait with grief that is not commonly acknowledged: They can both be tools for growth. Typically, grief throws down challenges you wonder whether you have the strength to bear, but which, over time, you can learn to live with, heal from, and even thrive because of.

Creativity, in a gentler fashion, can do the same. It will undoubtedly stretch and challenge you, but can be gentler than grief, because you can enjoy it! Choose an activity you love, are curious about, or have always wanted to try, and surrender to the healing power of creativity. Here are some key ways that creativity and a daily creative practice helped me and can help you.

This begins the creative section of this book. I have developed the formula for Creative Self-Empowerment. If you work through this book with diligence, focus, and flexibility I promise you will see positive changes in your life.

First look at yourself in the mirror and let your mind run free with your imagination, visualization and reflect on your story; your grief; and your pain. You may feel sad and lonely but placed the opposite images in your mind. Something of beauty.

These exercises will strengthen your Creative Brain.

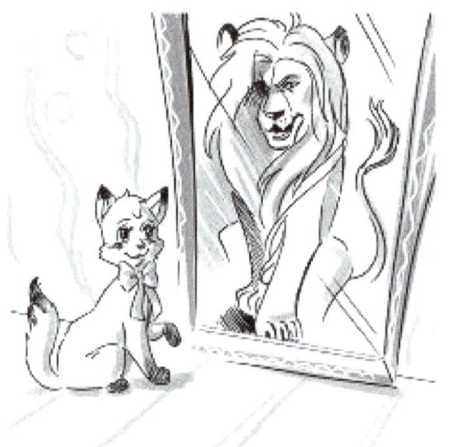

The left side of the brain is responsible for controlling the right side of the body. It also performs tasks that have to do with logic, such as in science and mathematics. On the other hand, the right hemisphere coordinates the left side of the body and performs tasks that have do with creativity and the arts. Take the Creative Self-Empowerment formula: **P= I M3H2=U X S** and visualize your creative self.

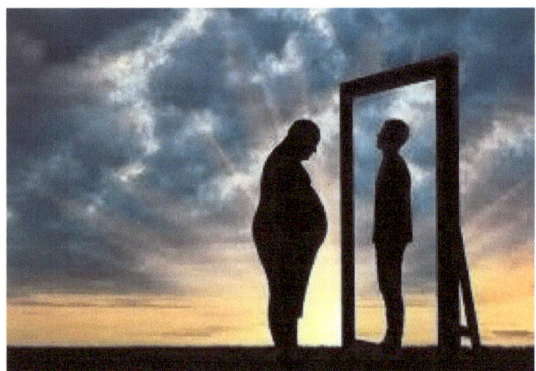

Creativity challenges us to look for and find beauty in our everyday life.

Page 30

The formula for creative self-empowerment

P= I M3H2=U x S

P – Power of Story

I – Insight

M3 – Movement, Mind Rest, and Mind Shift

H2 – Both Hands

U – Uniqueness of You

S - Spirituality

Creative self-empowerment involves a process of discovering the uniqueness of you through a creative therapeutic process. During this process it will make you feel more alive and learn how to delve deeper into your mental psychic (subconscious) and explore the inner workings of your mind. This is a dynamic and compelling process that will help you find your true and authentic self.

The Power of Story is to reflect on your life and working through the pain. Working through means uncovering and handling of your inner life memories, feelings, issues and concerns of deep pain. Through this discovery you will release the toxic thinking and craft a more hopeful and truthful narrative for yourself by building upon what was good in your past and breaking down and relinquishing what was not. You will reconstruct a more empowered self; working through allows you to manage and drawn energy from forces that once undermined you. You reconcile the past, so you can have a better future.

Insight involves an inner compass that is built upon self-knowledge. You cannot develop your own brand of custom designed self-mastery unless you have a deep awareness that tells you how and when to be strict with yourself and how and when to be lenient. Everyone has a unique receipt for self-mastery based on individual traits. When you understand yourself and follow your script outline you will have an easier time dealing with unexpected situation and getting along with others.

The Power of Story

Dr. David Krueger, my mentor has done extensive research on "The Neuroscience and Quantum Physics of Success: The Power of Story Breakthrough Strategies for Changing Life's Purpose, A Scientific System of Mind, Brain, and Behavior."

He states, by integrating sciences into creative expression, and co-constructing a new story for individuals, we shift:

- From problem to possibility
- From teaching to experiencing
- From telling to listening
- From observer to participant
- From educating to collaborating

Operating Systems

95% of our behaviors and core beliefs are pre-programmed in the unconscious mind.

We create two stories simultaneously:

- *The surface story* that we run our lives with conscious intentions and aspirations
- *The shadow story* that ghostwrites behaviors

Contributions from Psychology and Psychoanalysis

- Empathy: Listening position from inside one's experience
- Theory of mind: The ability to see the world from another person's vantage point
- Neutrality: Remaining equidistant from a one's dilemma, conflict, or ambivalence
- Learn from the old story: The past teaches the present
- When an emotion becomes a foreground issue it must be dealt with first
- The intersubjective third: Two people in a relationship create a third entity
- Regulating states of mind and managing emotions is a crucial success strategy
- Understanding our own dynamics and the dynamics of others
- Positive psychology and emotional intelligence move us from absence of disease to health
- Focus on the exception rather than the problem
- A Specific Application from Psychoanalysis to Mentoring and Change

- Transference: The repetitive ways of organizing current experiences based on past
- experiences
- Two kinds of memories activated in coaching: Explicit (factual) and implicit
- (procedural)
- Contributions from Neuroscience
- Mirror neurons: A function of networks in different parts of the brain that function
- reflect the behavior and feelings of others. Mirror neurons are instrumental into
- acquiring empathy, language, and social behavior.
- People have prior knowledge that affects how they hear and respond to new
- information
- The prior knowledge is physical, real, and persistent as a neuronal pathway in
- the brain
- If we ignore reality, it will get in the way of new information and change
- Partly because it is complex and personal and partly because it is subjective
- reality, people are not always aware of their prior knowledge.

Contributions from Quantum Physics

- Quantum physics helps us understand energy fields
- The activity of an observer affects what we observe.
- The power is in the focus
- The Law of Attraction
- Individual and collective energy fields: The unified field theory (Einstein)

Contributions from Social Psychology

The influence of social networks:

- If your immediate friends are obese, your risk of obesity is 45% higher
- If your friend becomes obese, it increases your chance of obesity by 57%
- If your friend's friends are obese, your risk is 25% higher
- This clustering of influence is caused by:
- Mirror neurons
- Induction
- Confounding effect

Contributions from Buddhism

- When one area of the brain is engaged, other components will be engaged
- Mind, brain, and body are a unified whole
- Meditation increases the number of neurons in brain regions that mediate attention, compassion, and empathy
- Meditation strengthens the immune system and improves psychological health

A Summary of Science Contributions

- Psychoanalysis addresses coming to an end of whole story, but not how to strategically create a new story.
- Quantum Physics recognizes the participation of the observer in the creation of reality, but omits motivation.
- Neuroscience illuminates workings of the conscious and unconscious mind, while disregarding the spirit.
- Psychology helps us understand the developmental role of effectiveness.

Collaborative, Contingent Conversations

The grief and the counseling process is a collaborative, contingent conversation:

- Collaborative: Both parties make contributions to an ongoing and contingent conversation.
- Contingent: There is no script, but what each person says is responsive to what the other just said.

Mentalization: A Theory of Mind

A theory of mind – attending to states of mind in others and ourselves – involves two concepts:

- Know yourself and your states of mind
- Understanding the difference of the mind and experiences of another person

We prompt insight and awareness in areas such as:

- Paying attention to new ways of thinking and behaving
- Focused attention on what is positive

- Avoiding exploration of motivation of why someone did something that didn't work
- Cultivate cognitive veto power on the negative and on the past
- Map new possibilities to reflect on expectations and values to align with goals
- Challenge and examine a person thinking that leads to a decision not to follow through on a commitment

Benefits of Mentalization Development

- Those with a stronger empathic ability can predict motives and actions of others, as well as understand and connect in a more comprehensive way
- Envisioning a future self-postpones impulses and engages productive activities

Mind Matters and Brain Business

Why do we resist change? Even changing a story that doesn't work?

- Part of the answer is in our minds
- Part of the answer is in our brains

New Narratives and Old Brains: The Need for Story

When a person tells and listens to stories it has an impact on:

- Blood pressure regulation
- Illness outcomes
- Attitude

We create our "selves" through narrative:

- Right brain: Intuition, emotion, creativity
- Left brain: Personal self-narrating thoughts and actions; the interpreter function

The Power of Story Exercises

The Us Story

Each important relationship becomes its own story, an *Us*. These practice exercises is to strengthen your Creative Brain by writing a script of your life that includes an important person, a family animal or anything that you love and value. A grief counselor and client illustrate the *Us* story.

The *Us* is a collaboratively constructed story between you and your counselor or grief support, and you establish who would take the lead in writing the script. You decided who would be the director that guide your story's artistic, and dramatic aspects to that fulfillment of your vision. The director has a key role giving direction when the story becomes painful and traumatic for the individual who is grieving. Directors need to be able to mediate differences in creative visions when you get stuck on verbalizing your feelings. There are many pathways in achieving this goal and our focus is to help you get unstuck by illustrating effective ways of using your Imagination, Creativity and the Power of Story. The Power of Story is writing a script on how you feel; expressing your emotions through words to see and understand what you are revealing through your story.

 A good director allows their actors outline a general plotline and let them improvise dialogue, while others control every aspect, and demand that the actors and crew follow instructions precisely. Some directors also write their own screenplays or collaborate on screenplays with long-standing writing partners. Some directors edit or appear in their films or compose the music score for their films. As the writer and director of your life it's you that will empower your story.

You as The Story Teller and Director

These Power of Story exercises will allow you to explore your own creativity. These daily practice of writing stories through pictures, images and imagination will create new neuron pathways for creativity. My mentor Dr. Krueger says, *"Creativity breeds Creativity."*

The Power of Story 1 - Vision
1) Write down your first thoughts when you see the following picture.
2) Write down everything you see in the picture, then let your spouse, partner, friend, parents, kids & others write down what they see. This will help you recognize and potentiate creativity.

3) Write the story of this picture with the focus on Vision and everything you see in the picture. There are no right or wrong answers and the goal is to develop your creative skills by writing a story. The writing of stories using a focus of Vision enhances the neurons in the Occipital Lobe which is the area for vision. The newer neurons you develop in your brain are analogous to lifting weights to strengthen your muscles; new neuron building is the mind and health fitness for a strong and healthy you.

Those who primarily process in a visual way record and construct pictures or internal images of their experiences they recall by snapping a picture into focus. Visual individuals will be inclined to say:

- Can you picture it?
- Bring this into focus.
- Mental image.
- I'd like to look at it
- I can see what you're saying
- It appears to me…
- It seems fuzzy to me.
- Short-sided

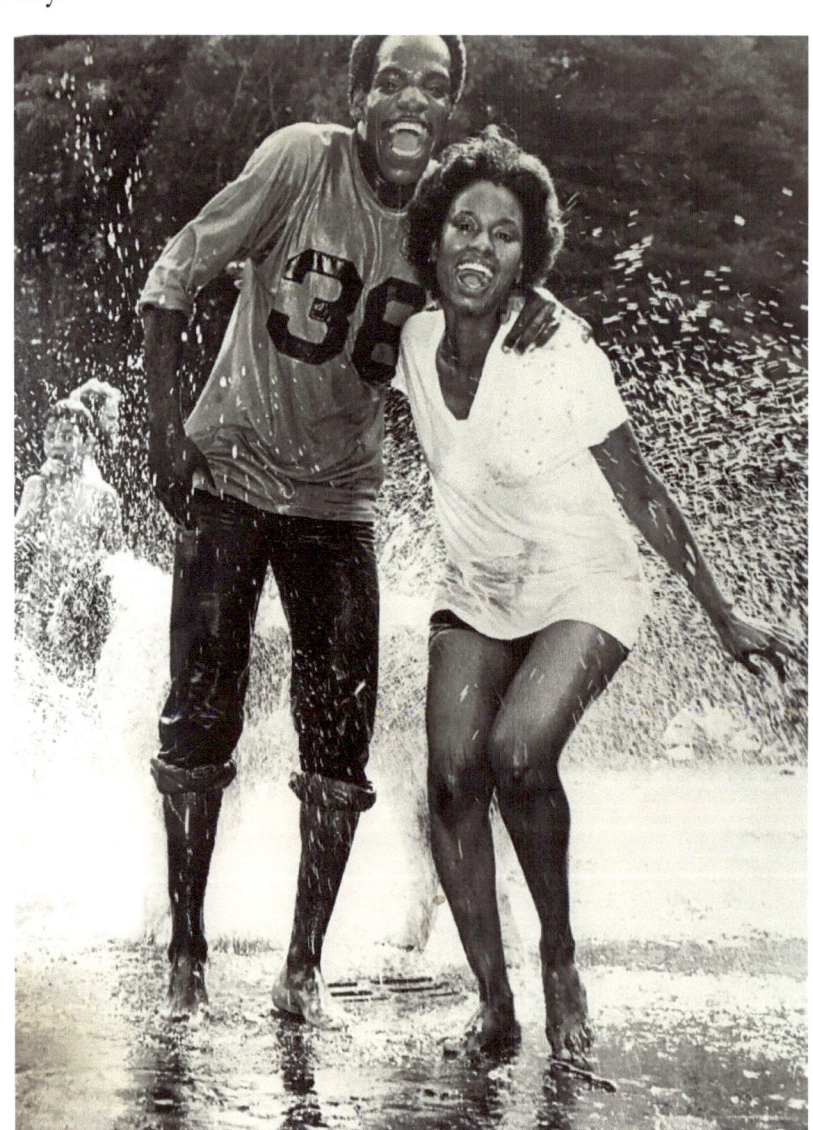

The Power of Story 2 – Auditory

How information is perceived and channeled is one element of a life story. Three fundamental representational systems elaborated in Neuro-Linguistic Programming based on the predominant representation channel include visual, auditory, and kinesthetic. How each person perceives, records, and recalls events depends on the predominant representational system used. These mind fitness exercises will do the following:

Update Your Operating System: Writing New Stories

The Brain's Story of Self

Listen to the story that the source inside you tells

- Tell your story the way you want it to be to actualize it
- Whatever you are living or experiencing is in response to the story you are
- telling. A new telling needs to align with who you are.
- When you practice your authentic story, your full energy and power becomes activated. You can keep telling and living a better story, no matter how good it is now.

First imagine yourself as this person and describe what you see with a focus on noise and sound. Can you hear the ripple sounds of the water? Is she splashing the water with the stick in her hand? Come on! Use your imagination and write the story.

Though not exclusive, an individual uses predominantly one representational mode. Those who take in information best through auditory presentation perceive experiences more in terms of sound and spoken word. They use phrases such as:

- I hear what you are saying
- It sounds good
- Within hearing
- I really want you to listen
- Tuned in
- Loud and clear

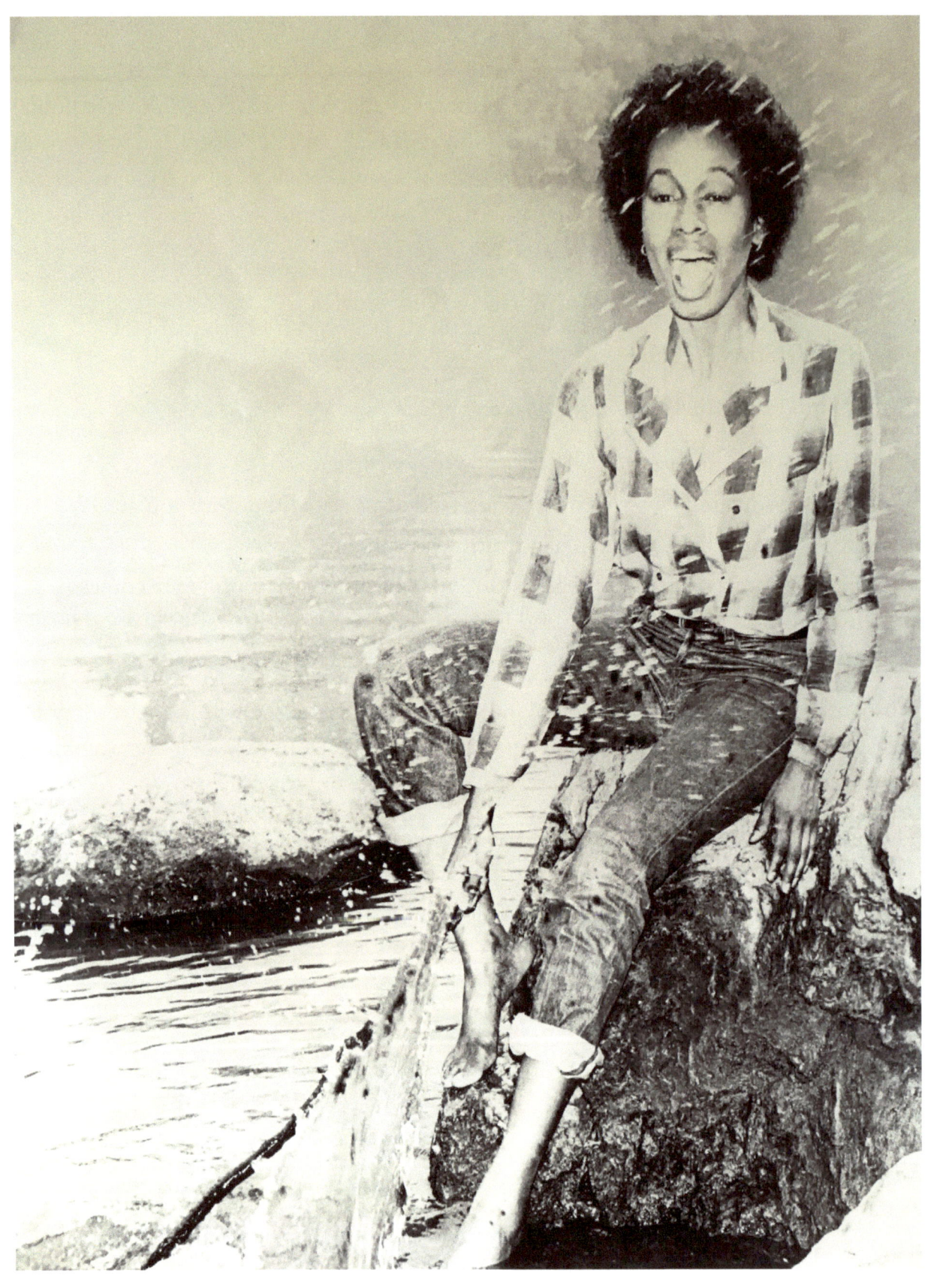

The Power of Story 3 – Kinesthetic

Kinesthetic individuals experience in a bodily way, and index information by sensation and feeling. Those more kinesthetic use sensory and bodily terms such as:

- I need to grasp that
- To be more in touch with…
- Come to grips with
- Hand in hand
- Hold on
- Hold that though
- Able to get a handle on it
- Start from scratch
- I'll walk you through this
- It slipped through my hands

What does this picture say to you? Write her story. Do you feel any empathy or compassion for this person? Developing empathy and establishing rapport with another can be facilitated by awareness of the other's primary representational system.

Neuro-linguistic program researchers and practitioners have distilled some basic principles of recognizing the model and using it to facilitate communication.

- Recognize the predominant channel of processing information for yourself and your client, patient, and partner: auditory, visual, or kinesthetic.
- Respect the other person's model of the world, of perceiving and processing information along one of the three representational systems. One is not better than the other, just different.
- The observational skills of the type and meaning of communication is a necessary component of emotional intelligence.

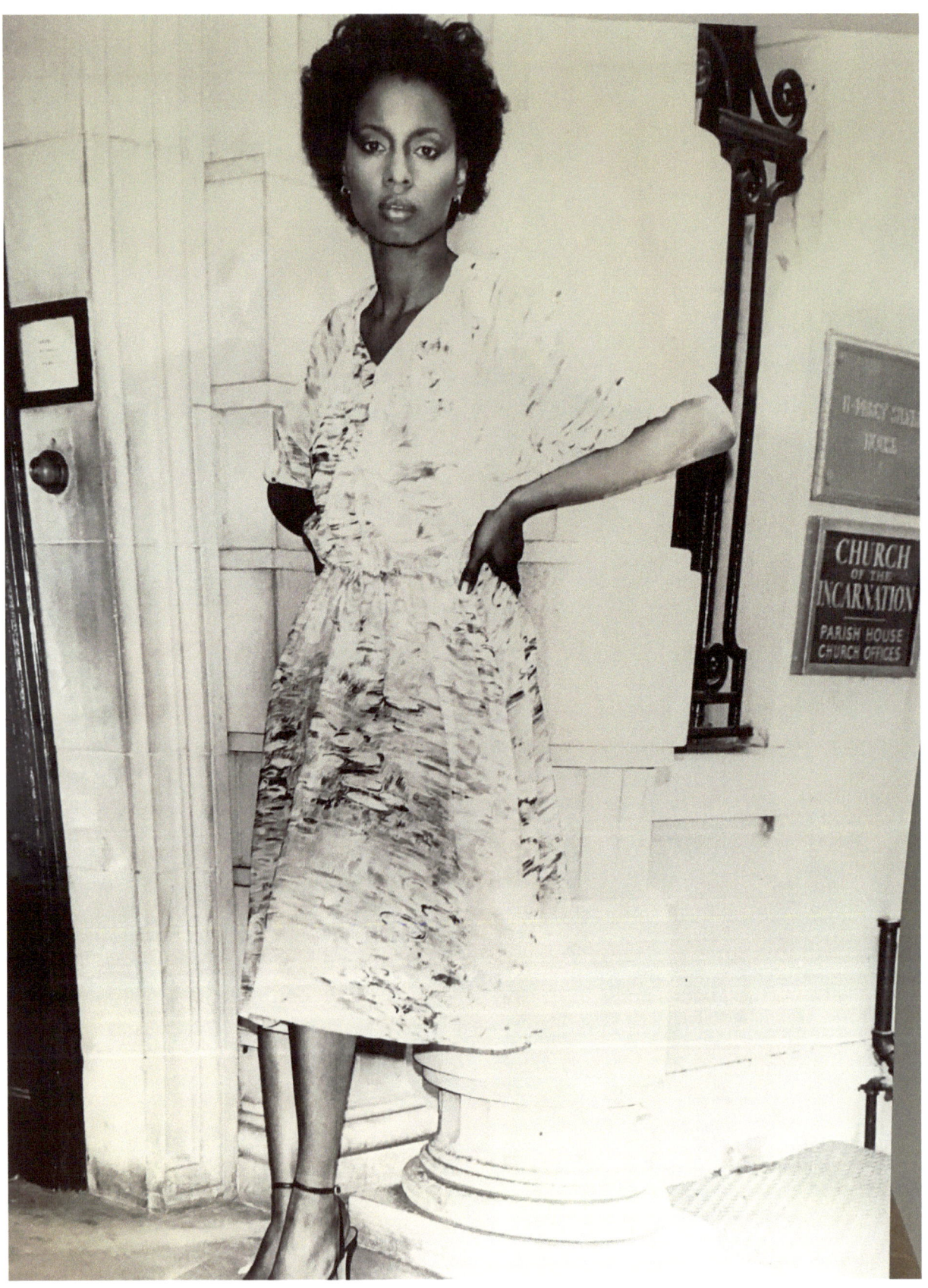

My Creative Writing Story -

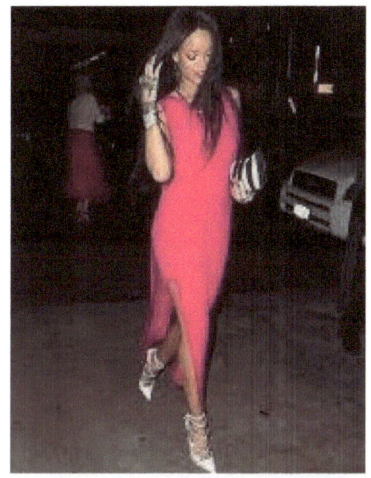
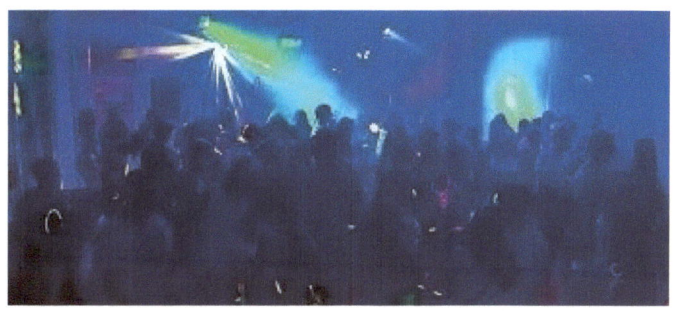

The Cafe and My LONG Pink Silky Dress

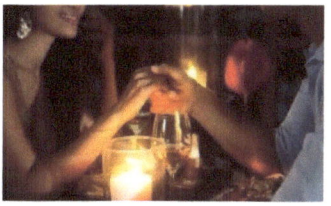

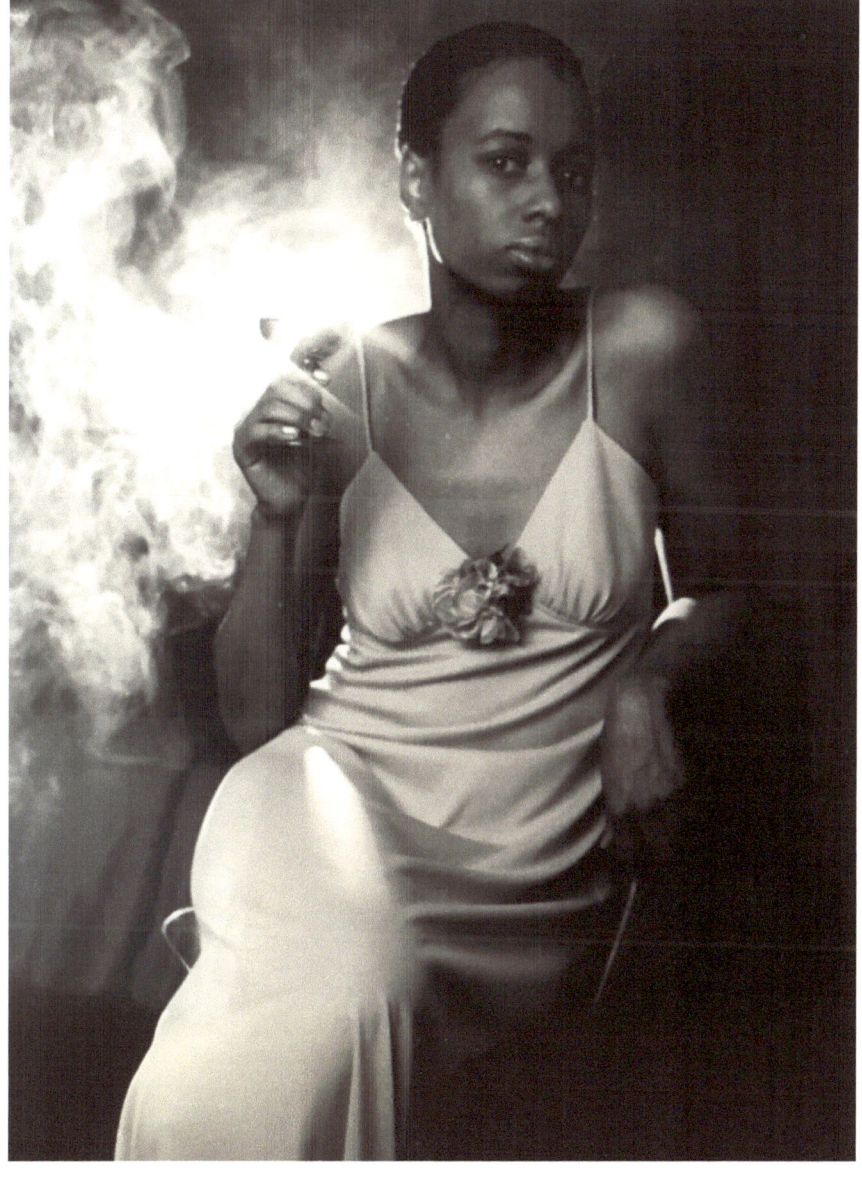

I'm what you considered a "Good Girl." I've never smoked, rarely drink and no drug use. Today, I'm a middle-aged woman and I've only known one man in my life. I reflect on a make-believe story, a woman in her 20s, who has lived a sheltered life, lonely and with few friends. I walk to my closet and see this sexy silky long pink dress that I've never wore because no one has asked me out on a date. I put it on and began to walk from my home to an unfamiliar neighborhood. It is very lively, people walking in a hurry, talking loudly and several glanced over at me with a smile. It's a warm beautiful day but the sun is setting, kids are playing in an open fire hydrant with the gush of water coming out. I'm careful not get any water on my dress. I continue to walk, feeling full of energy and a sense of freedom. As I pass this night club I hear the song, "My Cherie Amour," I'm familiar with the song but it doesn't sound like the singer Stevie Wonder. In fact, it's a woman voice and she's singing a French version of the song…I like it! The beats and music draw me into the club, and I sit down on the stool; and the bartender asked, "What can I get you?" I just blurted out a glass of champagne. I'm feeling freer and freer in this smoke-filled room and a tall man approach me…. what happens next!

This is an example of practicing writing stories with plots, subplots and themes. This neuron building exercise with daily practice and focus will help you solve your personal and professional problems. It builds your faith and confidence in all areas of your life. Have your ever heard the saying, *Faith is like a muscle, you must work it to see results?*

The Shaman and I

How to regain the proper alignment of mind, body and spirit

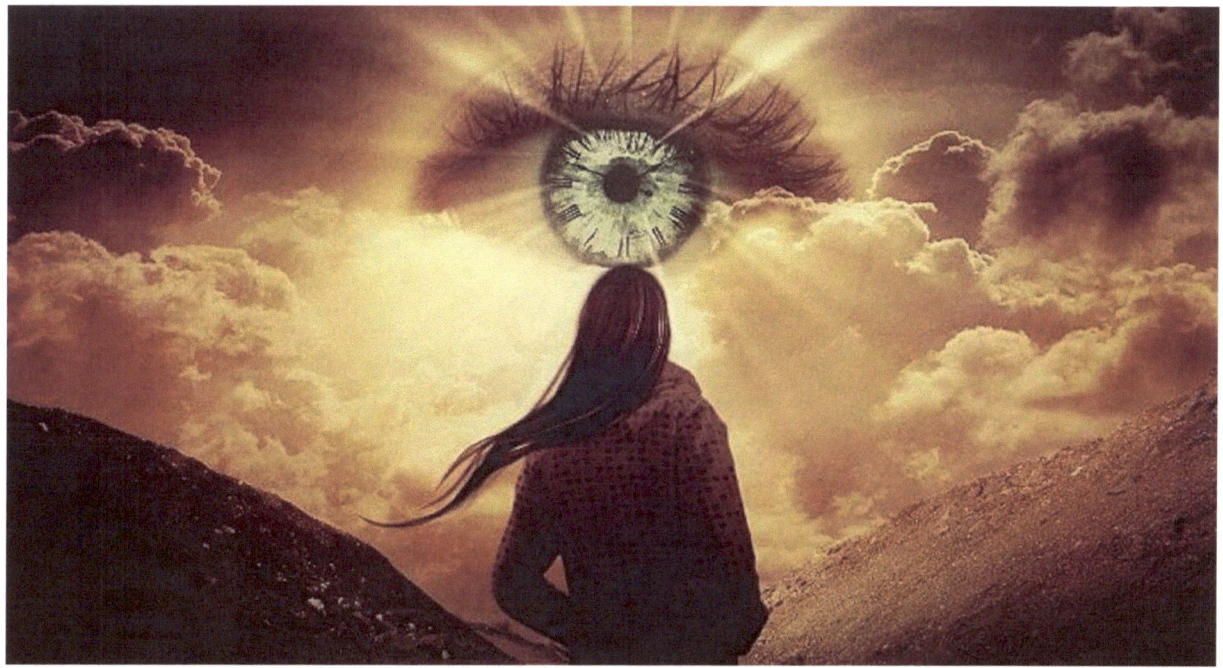

I was both fortunate and unfortunate enough to be a child of mixed heritage. My father was a Sioux Indian and my mother African American. My childhood was sandwich between two conflicting cultures. I experienced the richness and sadness of both. My American Indian heritage taught me to respect nature and placed a great emphasis on the harmony of mind, body and spirit. I had trouble trying to reconcile both cultures during my early adolescence. This caused me to resent both. I discussed these feelings with my parents. They took me to see an elderly Shaman, who explained that I was out of balance with the forces inside of me. He interpreted my feelings of emptiness and isolation as an absence of presence. He told me that I needed to restore harmony within my inner self. He informed me to stop trying to understand what I was feeling and just feel. He guided me through the proper process of meditation. He instructed me on how to find that special place, away from the flurry of my disharmonious thoughts, with his guidance I was able to experience stillness and peace. I am grateful to this

wonderful healer for teaching me a technique that I have used for many years to regain the proper alignment of mind, body and spirit. There is a thin line between normal and abnormal behavior; between psychiatric illness and somatic illness. We are all plagued by personal demons

Motivating Yourself

You're going to embark on a wonderful journey that will bring positive changes in all areas of your life, but you must do the work! The tools in this book I have used for years and they work! The author and minister Mike Murdock states, *"You will never leave where you are until you decide where you would rather be.*

Grief could be a desire and motivator destroyer. We have all wake up in the morning after a death of a loved one and loss our desire in work and accomplishing our daily duties…the Dream of a beautiful life is gone. I know, it happened to me. I've had many family deaths over the last few years plus my personal heartbreak experience but when I used these tools it re-ignited my passion for life.

Many people with great potential and great dreams have lost their motivation to achieve them. When you drive by a graveyard, remember this…many are inside those graves with buried dreams, buried treasures, buried potential…that never was fulfilled…because they lost their motivation.

Motivate yourself toward imagining, visualizing, breath work and exercising daily. A spiritual framework or positive affirmation for the circumstances of your life to change is your anchor for the best and worst of times.

Let's begin with the tools to Master a Successful You!

Imagination

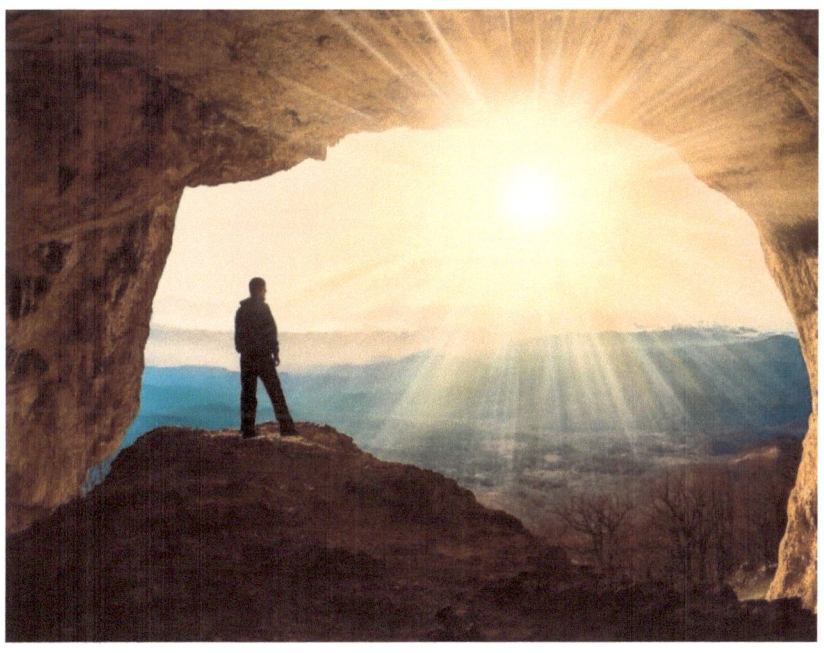

Imagination Is the Key to Your Future

You will always move in the direction of your strongest and most dominant thought. Your imagination is an invisible machine inside your mind that creates pictures of something in your future. Pictures of those things you desire. As human beings we are blessed with a Powerful organ, *The Brain* and it partner *The Mind.* There are two major functions of your mind. One is your memory, the other is your imagination. Your memory will photograph, file and replay pictures of your past. Your imagination, on the other hand, creates and replays pictures of things you want to happen in your future.

The Imagination Exercise – The Hot Air Balloon

This exercise will help you to relieve your fear and anxiety. It will enhance the creative side of your brain and with neuron building releasing the good hormones to make you relieve stress and feel good.

Imagined you're at a balloon show, sitting around with family and friends having a great time. A close friend asked you to go on a hot balloon ride. This will be your first time and you're reluctant, but he convinced you to go. Imagine yourself of being there and take note of your feelings and emotions. How do you feel? Anxious? Fearful or Excited!

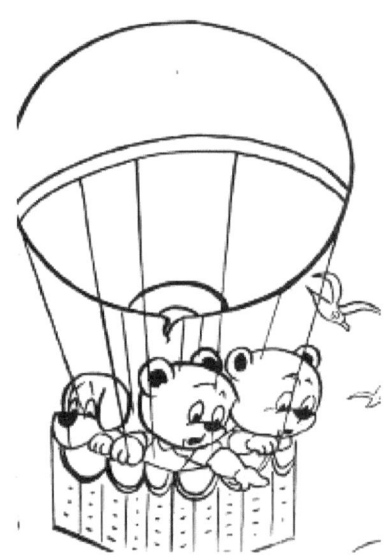

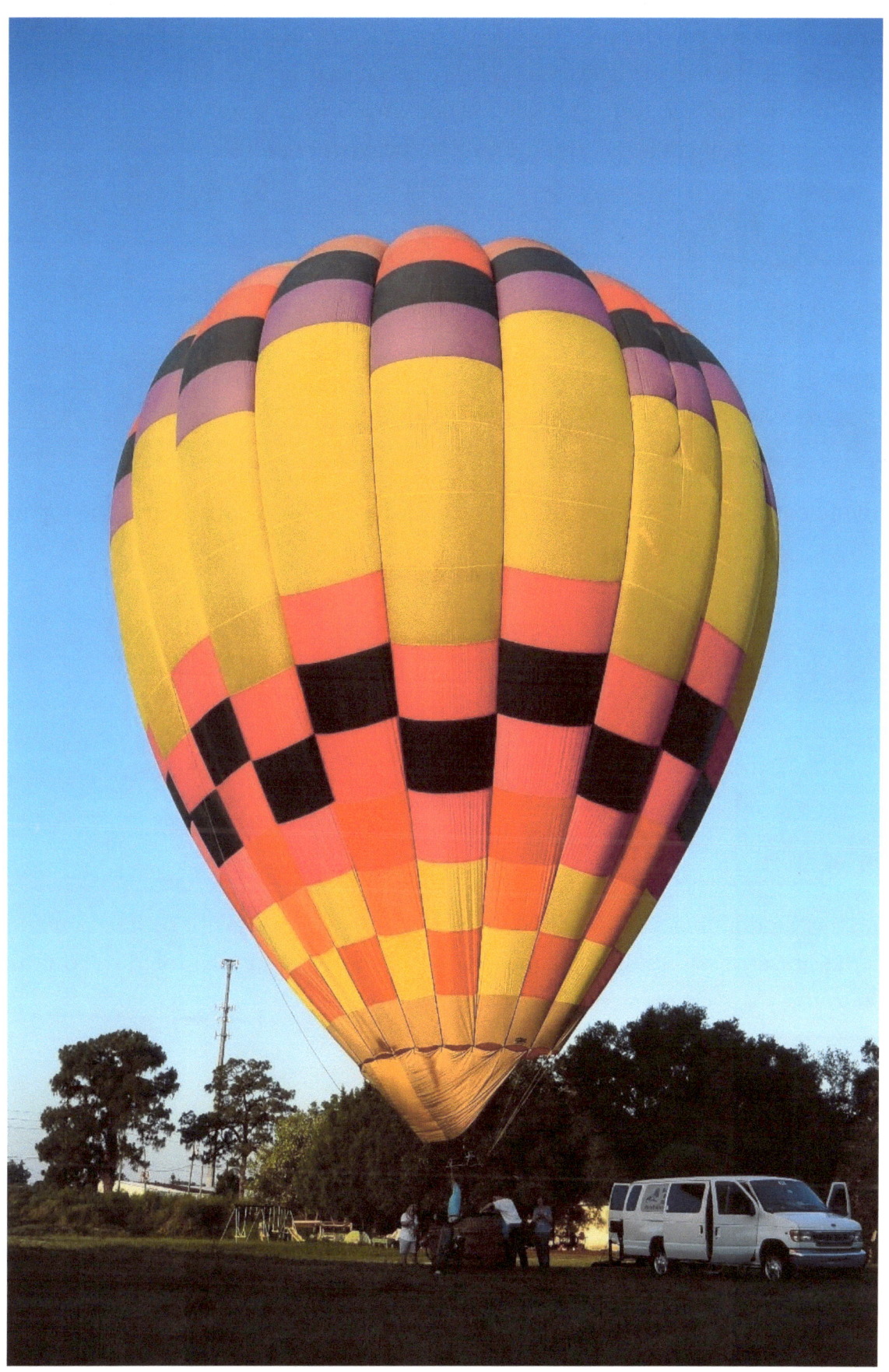

Imagine you've asked your friend, *"How does a hot-air balloon work?"* He replies, "The hot air trapped inside the balloon is heated up by a burner, making it less dense than the air outside." Imagine that the fear is building inside of you to take a hot air balloon ride, but it is too late! It's a windy day and the balloon begins to rise….

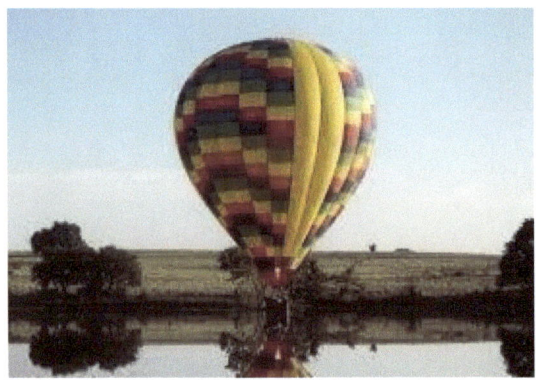

Your friend controls the balloon's altitude by releasing hot air from a vent at the top of the balloon….and it gets higher!

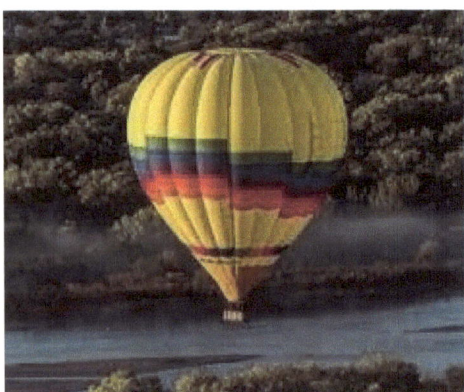

Imagine the wind hitting against your face. You begin to feel a sense of freedom and joy. As the sunset, it's a beautiful picture and take a snap shot in your mind so you can hold on to it.

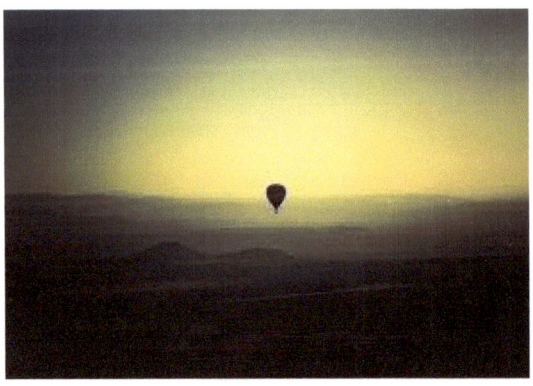

This new photograph will placed you in a different state of mind and creating new energy and motivation.

The balloon has taken you higher and higher physically and mentally.

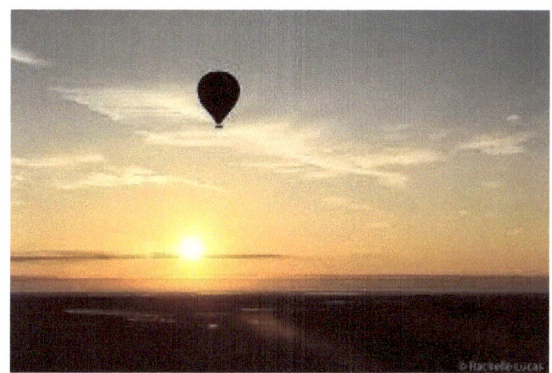

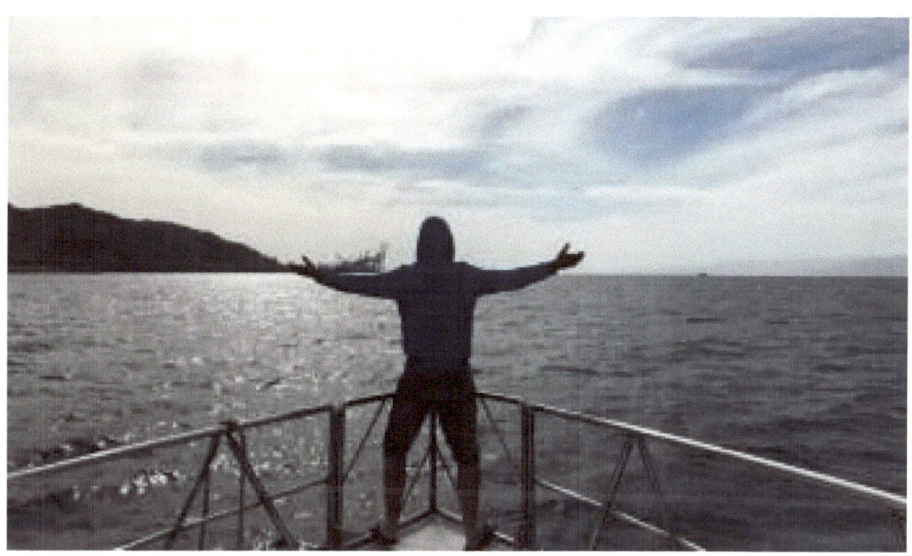

YOU MADE IT!

Your imagination can be your friend when you trust and believe in it. It can also be your enemy if your thoughts are of fear, lack of confidence and low self-esteem. It is your responsibility to protect your mind and imagination. Thoughts will invade your imagination from almost everywhere. Thoughts of fear and unbelief are invaders of the mind, but we are in control of our mind, body and spirit; and must protect it.

Visualization = Goal Setting

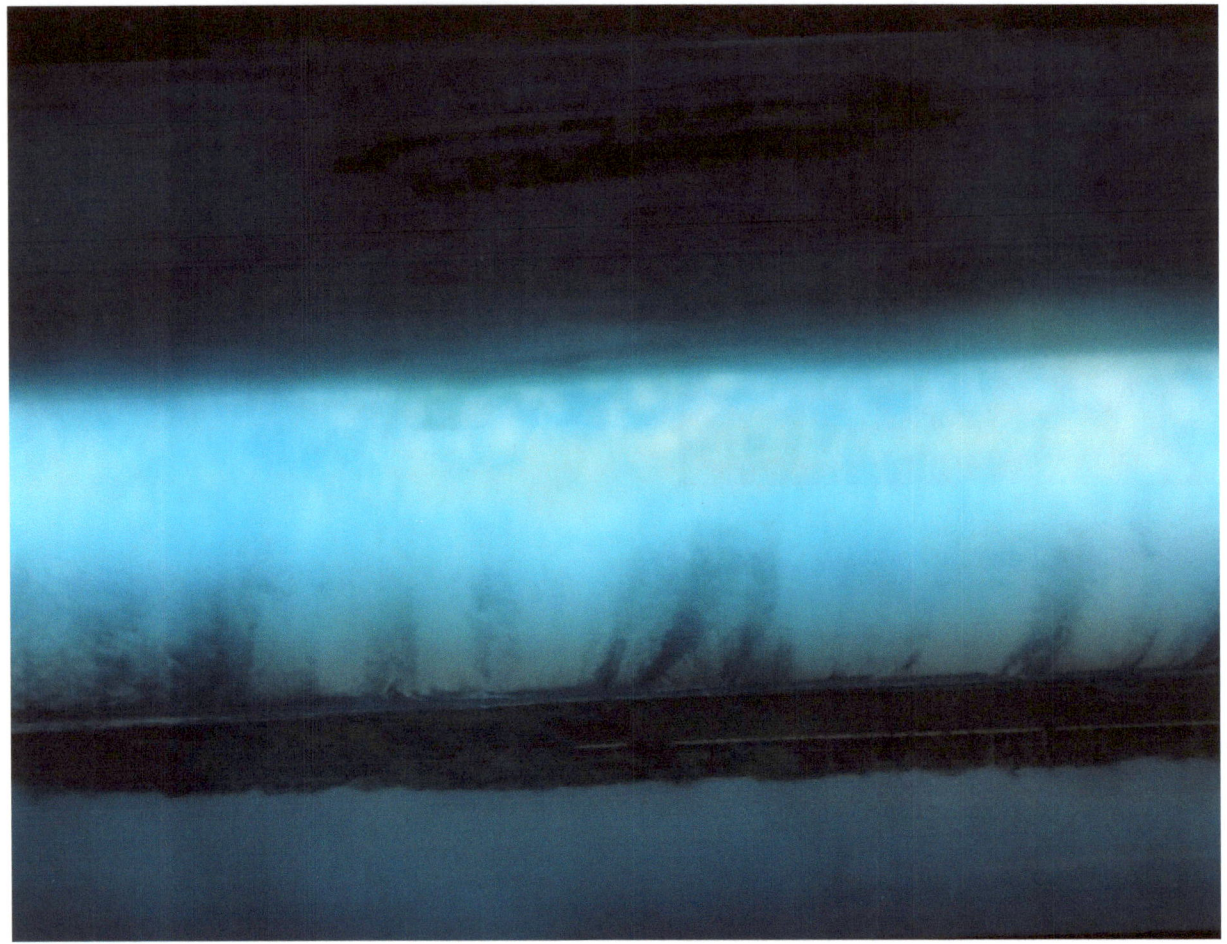

Visualization is the focus form of imagination because your thoughts are fixed on a specific goal. Your visualization will be anything that you will in your mind. But it is a basic law in achieving great successes. Your life will always move in the direction of your dominating thought. Your vision is the workshop of your mind. You can *Dream*, *Design* and *Determine* what you want to happen in your life. Whatever dominates your vision today will very likely be experience in your life tomorrow.

The Waterfall Exercise

Intention refers to the goal that you want to manifest in your life. Everything we do has an underlying intention, whether we are conscious of it or not, and we use it to determine what we really want to focus on: money, financial success, power, peace, romance, etc. Therefore, the first step is Relaxation which is the easiest way to reduce stress. Deep relaxation promotes neurological and cardiovascular health, and it also improves attentiveness, alertness, memory function and social awareness. It turns down the activity in the emotional brain, where anxiety, doubts, and uncertainty are always on the verge of derail your intention and goals.

- Look at the waterfall
- Breathe in slowly through your nose and exhale (3 times)
- Visualize yourself observing the waterfalls, hearing a cascade of water falling from an unknown height
- With each phase of waterfall see yourself getting closer which represent getting closer to your heart's desire or goal.
- As you walk toward the waterfall you hear the sound of turbulence which align with struggles that you may encounter to reach your goal.
- Breath in and out (3 times) and look closer at the picture…what do you see? A patch of greenery which align with something positive.
- Visualize the streams becoming wider and shallower just above waterfalls due to flowing over the rock shelf, and there is a deep area just below that waterfall because of the kinetic energy of the water hitting the bottom.
- The kinetic energy represents motivation to keep going and not give up on your dreams.

Desire and vision are the dominant seed for change. Your desires and vision are always more motivating than your needs. It was desire that inspired the Wright brothers to fly. It was desire that motivated Thomas Edison to persist through 10,000 experiments that failed before perfecting the light bulb. Don't Give Up!

To hear the actual sound of the waterfalls, go to www.audreygriefexpressionist.com and click on the vision tab.

Meditation = The Language of Love, Peace, and Mind Power

Buddha was asked: "What you gained from Meditation?" He replied: "Nothing." "However," Buddha said, "Let me tell you what I lost: Anger, Anxiety, Depression, Insecurity, Fear of Old Age and Death."

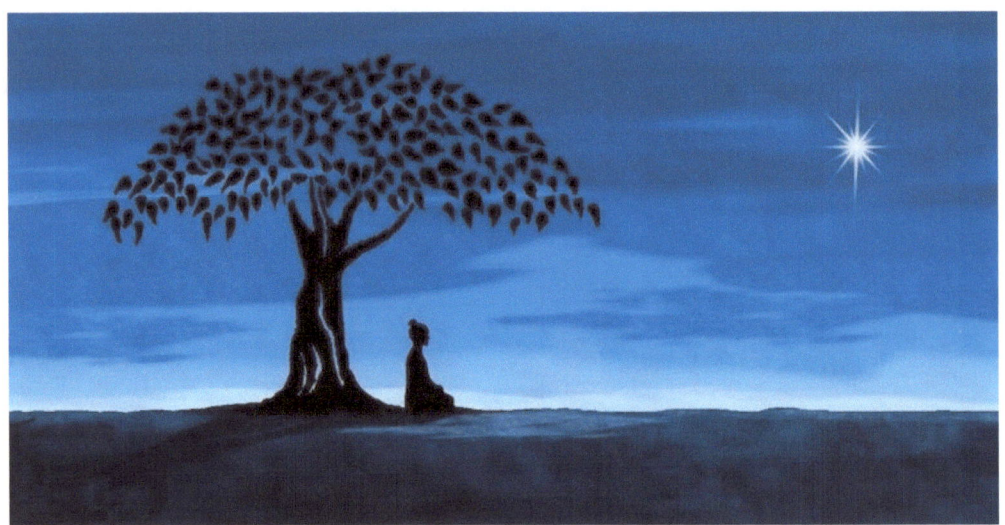

Meditation is the *Expression of Love* for yourself. Why? With love of self you place focus on inner peace and self-awareness. This *Power of Self* allows your mind, thoughts and ideas flow into the *Love of Living*, improving your quality of life, stress relief and an inner and outer guide of self-empowerment. The stillness and peace of conflict allows you to think clearer and relaxed your mind, body and spirit axis bringing a harmonious and balance state of mind.

A Ball of Confusion State of Mind

Do you feel confused in your thinking?

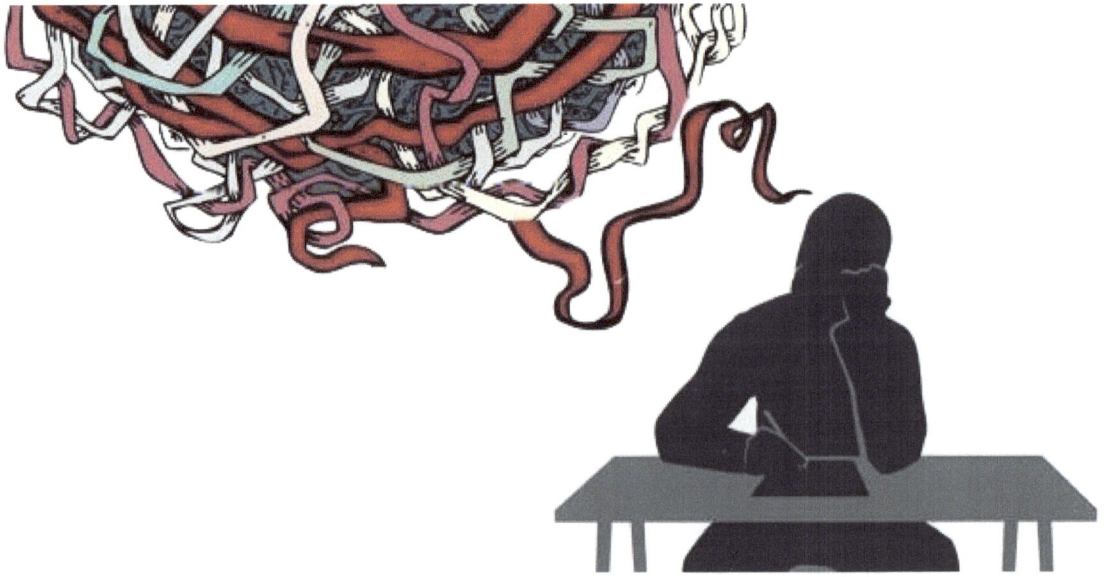

Do you feel so stressed you can't decide which way to go or what to do?

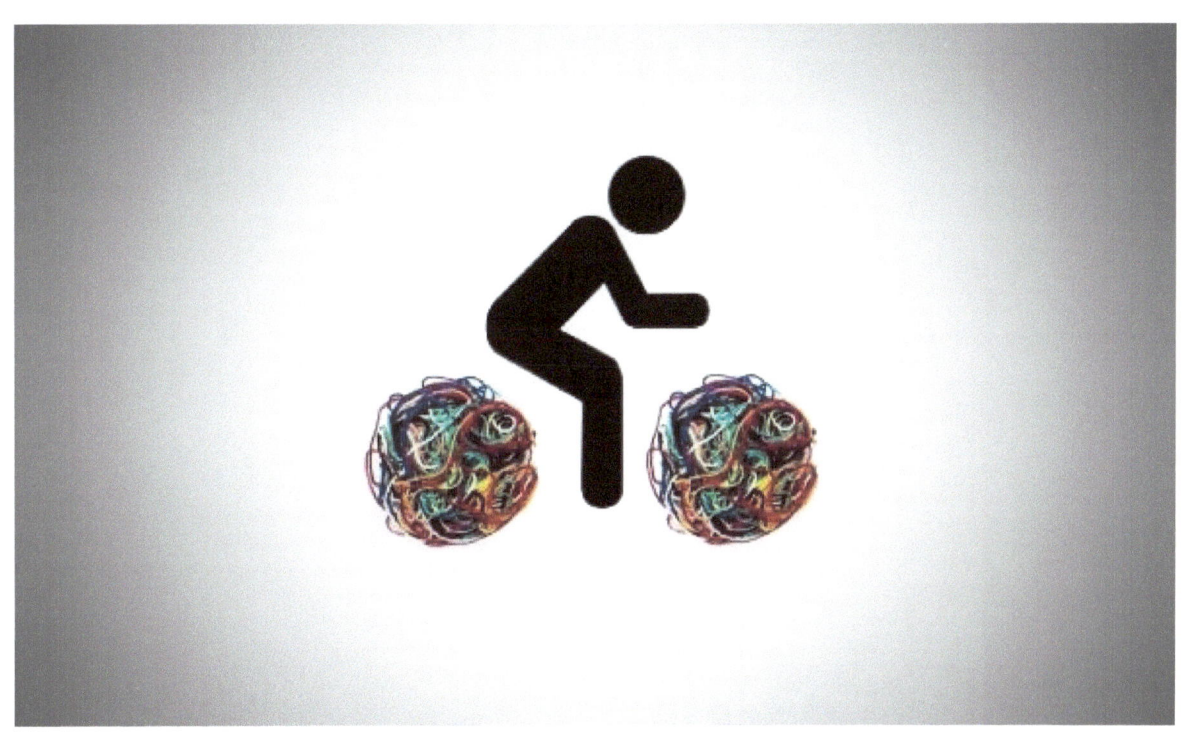

Meditation with Deep Breathing and Affirmations Brings It All Together

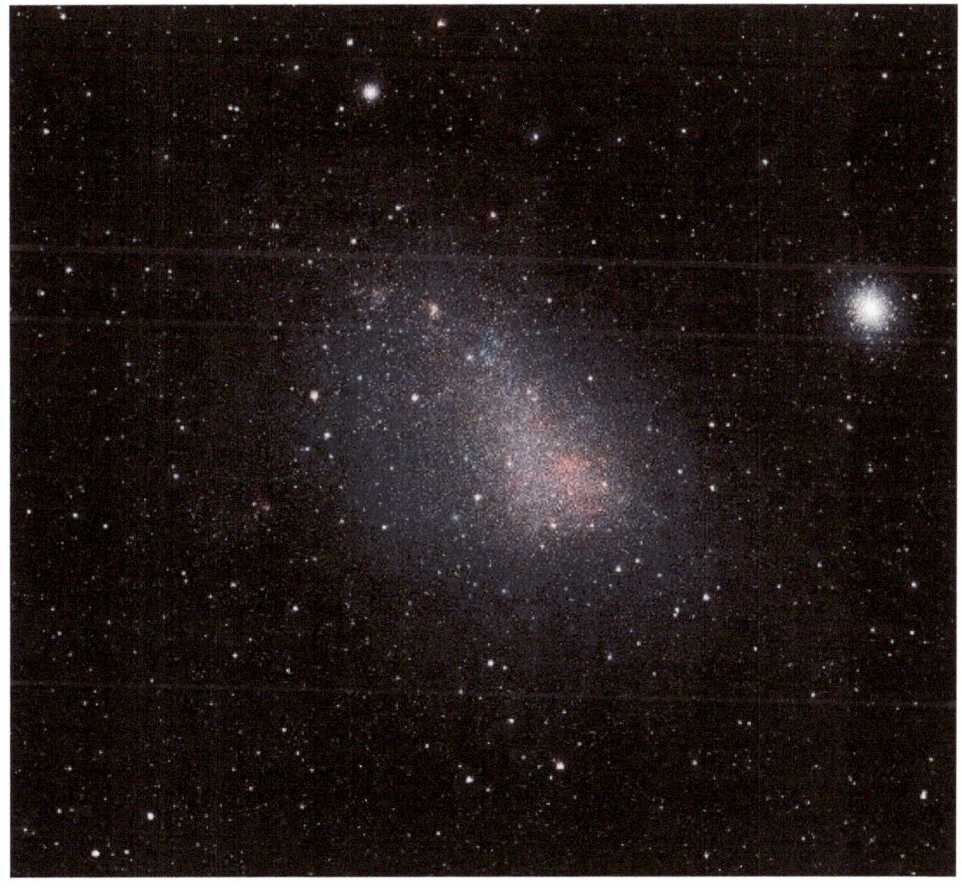

Cool Breathing

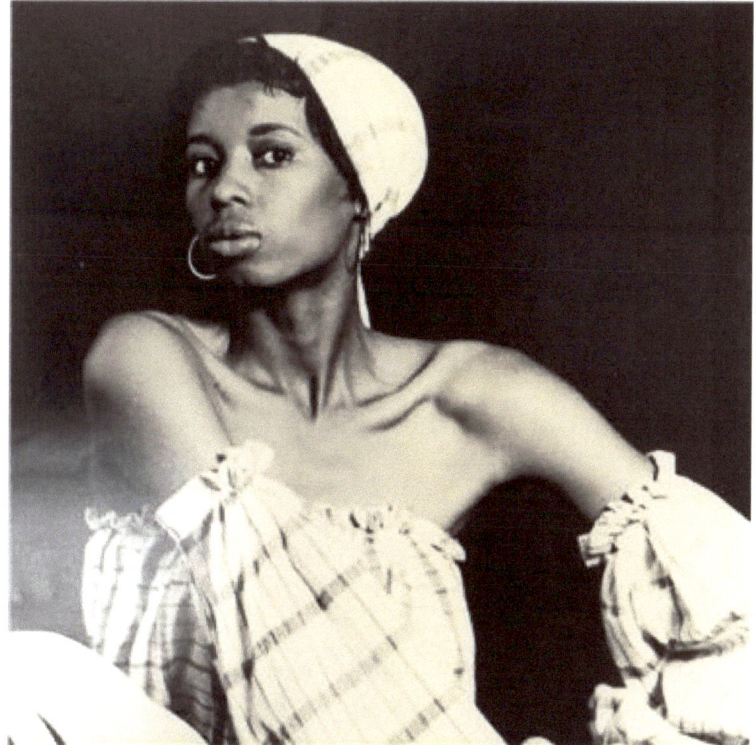

Why Is Breathing Cool?

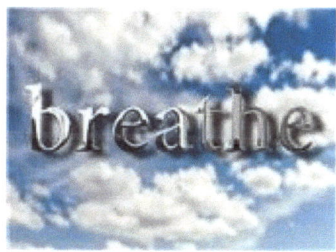

Because It Keeps Us Alive!

There are several reasons why breathing is important. First, it's the key to every human being's survival to sustain life. Our breathing system supplies oxygen to vital organs of the body, so they can function properly and keep us alive. Secondly, breathing is one means by which we get rid of waste products and toxins from the body.

Why Oxygenation of The Body Is So Vital?

Oxygen is the most vital nutrient for our bodies. It is essential to maintain the integrity of the brain, nerves, glands and internal organs. We can do without food for weeks and without water for days, but without oxygen, we will die within a few minutes. If the brain does not get proper supply of this essential nutrient, it will result in the degradation of all vital organs in the body.

The brain is the most important organ in the body and it requires more oxygen than any other organ. If it doesn't get enough, the result is mental sluggishness, negative thoughts, depression and, eventually, vision and hearing decline. Our seniors, and those whose arteries are clogged, often become senile and vague because oxygen to the brain is reduced. They get irritated more quickly.

Poor oxygen intake affects all parts of the body. The oxygen supply is reduced to all parts of the body as we get older due to poor lifestyle. Many people need reading glasses and suffer hearing decline in old age. These are some examples of poor oxygenation in the body:

- When an acute circulation blockage deprives the heart of oxygen, a heart attack is the result. If this occurs to the brain, the result is a stroke.

- For a long time, lack of oxygen has been considered a major cause of cancer. Even as far back as 1947, work done in Germany showed that when oxygen was withdrawn, normal body cells could turn into cancer cells.

Similar research has been done with heart disease. It showed that lack of oxygen is a major cause of heart disease, stroke and cancer. The work done at Baylor University in the USA (reference link) has shown that you can reverse arterial disease in monkeys by infusing oxygen into the diseased arteries.

Thus, oxygen is very critical to our well-being, and any effort to increase the supply of oxygen to our body and especially to the brain will pay rich dividends. Breathing correctly is very important for adequate oxygenation throughout the body. In my upcoming *"Cool Breathing book and CD"* I share the 8 effective breathing techniques that I have developed and perfected. These breathing exercises are particularly important for people who have sedentary jobs and spend most of the day in offices. Their brains are oxygen starved and their bodies are just 'getting by'. They feel tired, nervous and irritable and are not very productive. On top of that, they sleep badly at night, so they get a bad start to the next day continuing the cycle.

Oxygenation of the Body Purifies the Blood Stream

One of the major secrets of vitality and rejuvenation is a purified blood stream. The quickest and most effective way to purify the blood stream is by taking in extra supplies of oxygen from the air we breathe. The breathing exercises described below are the most effective methods ever devised for saturating the blood with extra oxygen.

Oxygen burns up the waste products (toxins) in the body, as well as recharging the body's batteries (the solar plexus). In fact, most of our energy requirements come not from food but from the air we breathe.

By purifying the blood stream, every part of the body benefits, as well as the mind. Your complexion will become clearer and brighter and wrinkles will begin to fade away. In short, rejuvenation will start to occur.

The Benefits of Proper Breathing

- Lower your stress levels
- Maintain a stable blood pressure to effectively reduce the damaging effects of stress
- Keeps you relaxed and free from anxiety

How to Start Benefiting from Effective Breath Work

Start with 'deep-breathing'. Here's a simple-yet-effective step-by-step guide by Harvard Medical School to show you how to practice deep breathing.

1) Find a quiet, comfortable place to sit or lie down.
2) Close your eyes, sit comfortably with your back straight and take a normal breath.
3) Now take a deep breath lasting 5-6 seconds. Breathe in slowly through your nose, let your chest and lower belly expand as you fill your lungs with the air. Let your abdomen expand fully.
4) Hold on to it for just a few seconds.
5) Now breathe out SLOWLY through your mouth, again lasting within 5-6 seconds.
6) Continue the process. And now try to observe the rhythm of your body as you go about breathing. Put one hand on your abdomen, just below your belly

button. Feel your hand rise about an inch each time you inhale and fall an inch each time you inhale and fall an inch each time you exhale. Remember to relax your belly so that each inhalation expands it fully.

7) Repeat the process. Only, now you should blend deep breathing with something that will help you relax and focus. It can be an image (the beach or hiking), or a scene from your favorite movie or perhaps even a quote or phrase.

Deep breathing, at first, can be quite challenging and you may not feel that it is very relaxing. But with some practice (just like riding a bicycle) you will get used to it and it will get easier from then on.

Eight Effective Breathing Techniques

Sit comfortably in a chair or on the floor with loose clothing and follow each simple breathing technique.

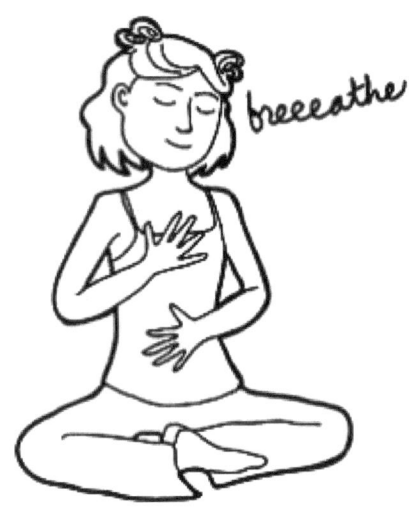

normal breathing

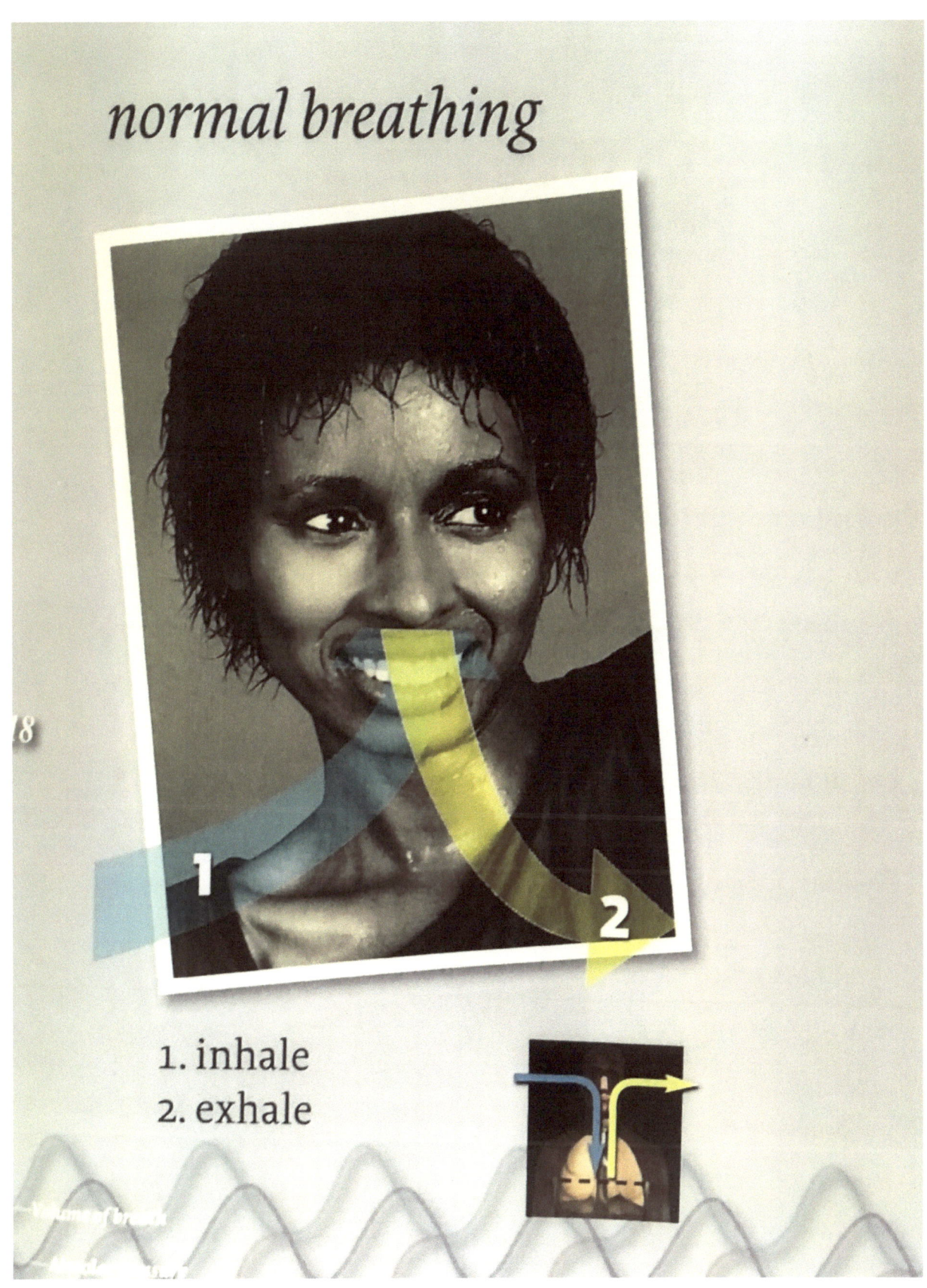

1. inhale
2. exhale

reverse breathing

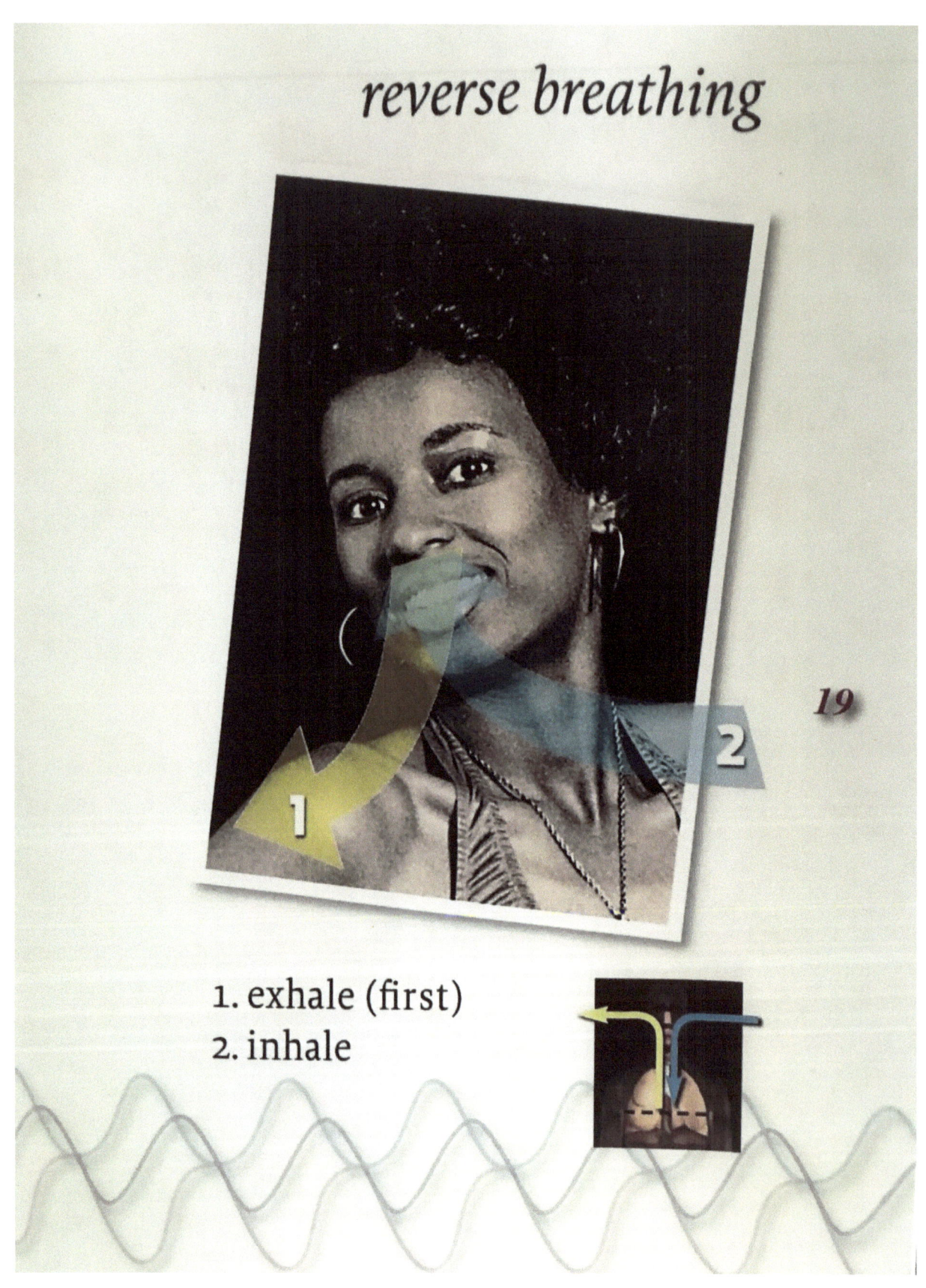

1. exhale (first)
2. inhale

deep breathing

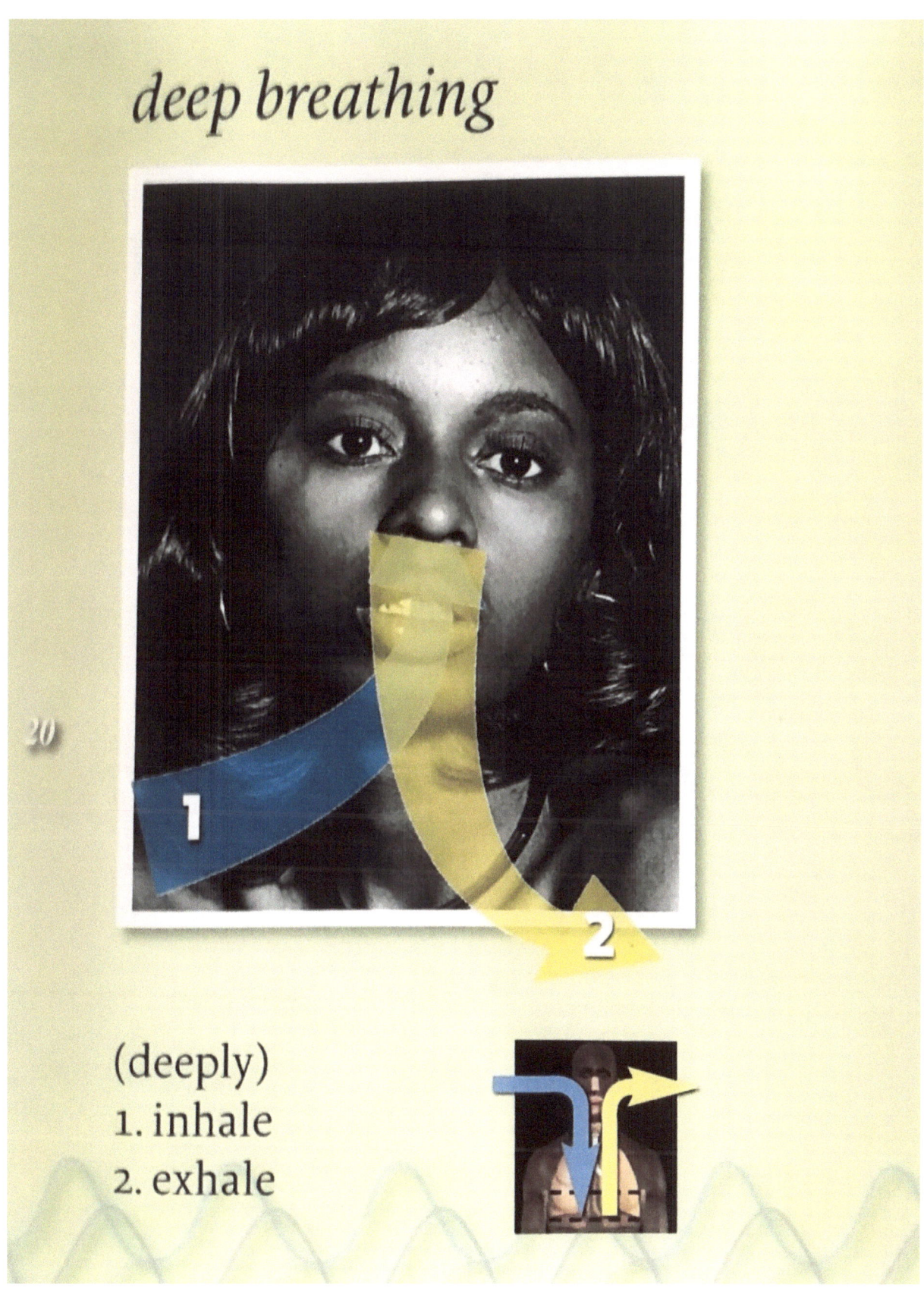

(deeply)
1. inhale
2. exhale

additional exhalation

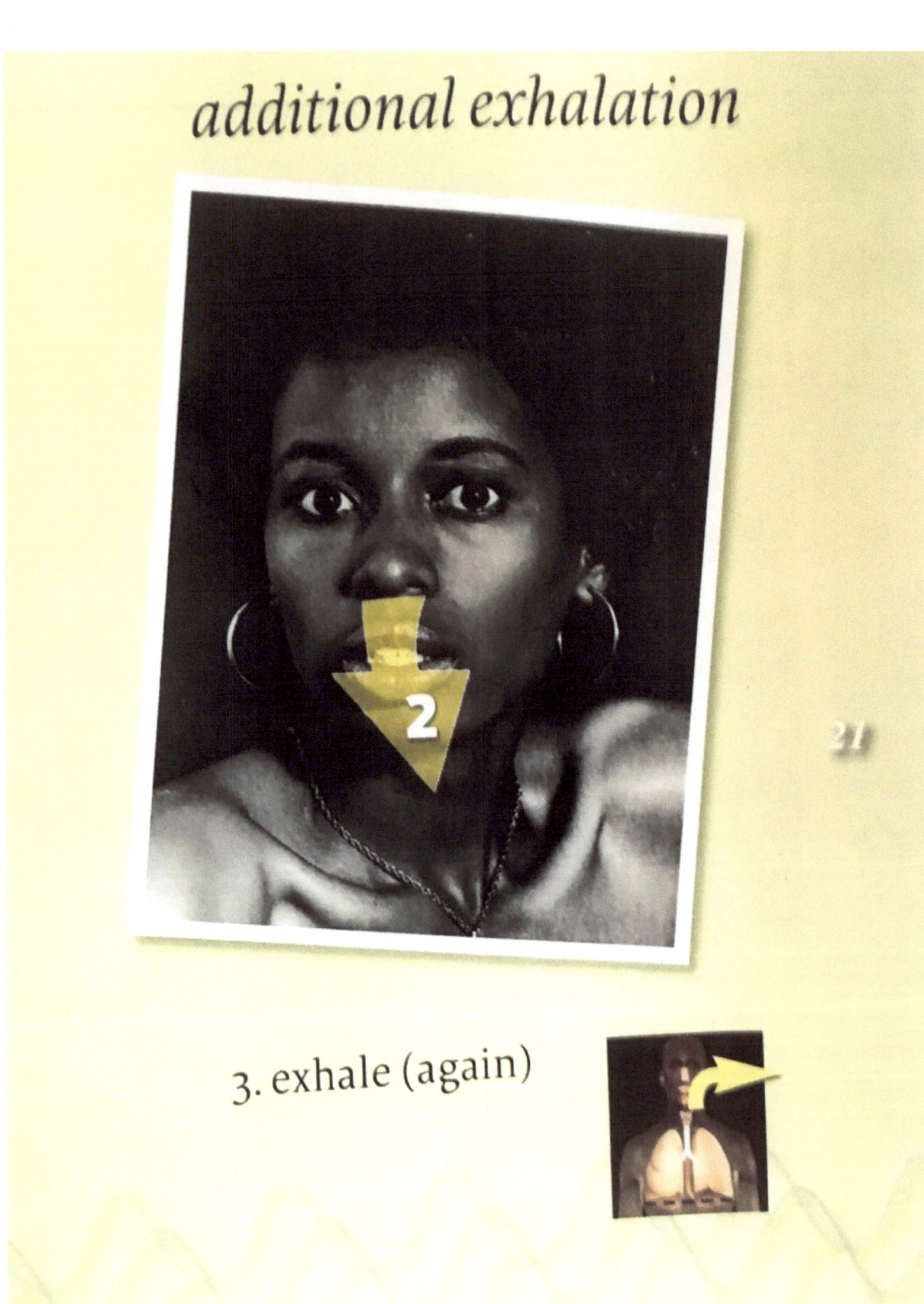

3. exhale (again)

rapid breathing

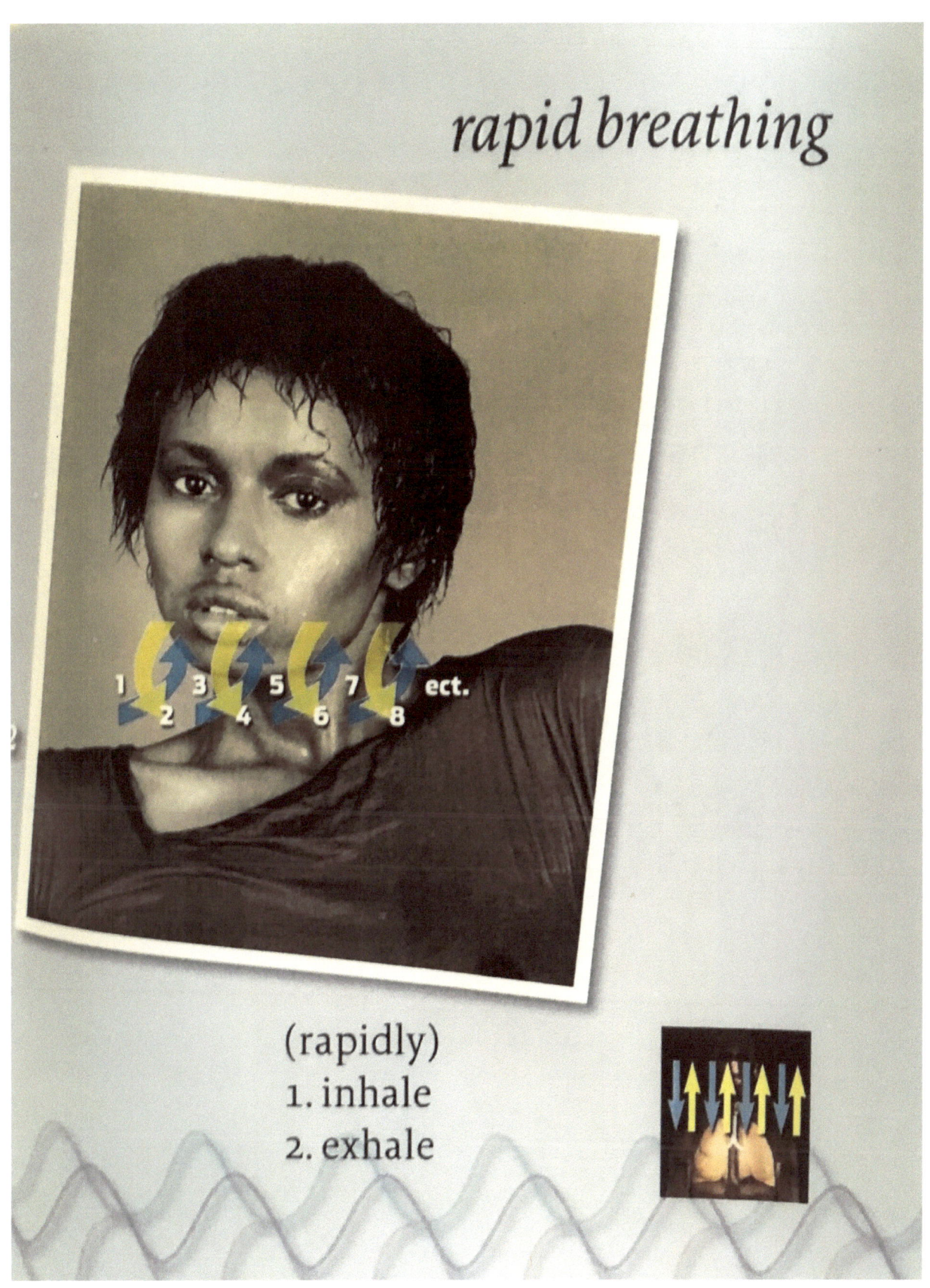

(rapidly)
1. inhale
2. exhale

count "1-2-3-4-" HOLD

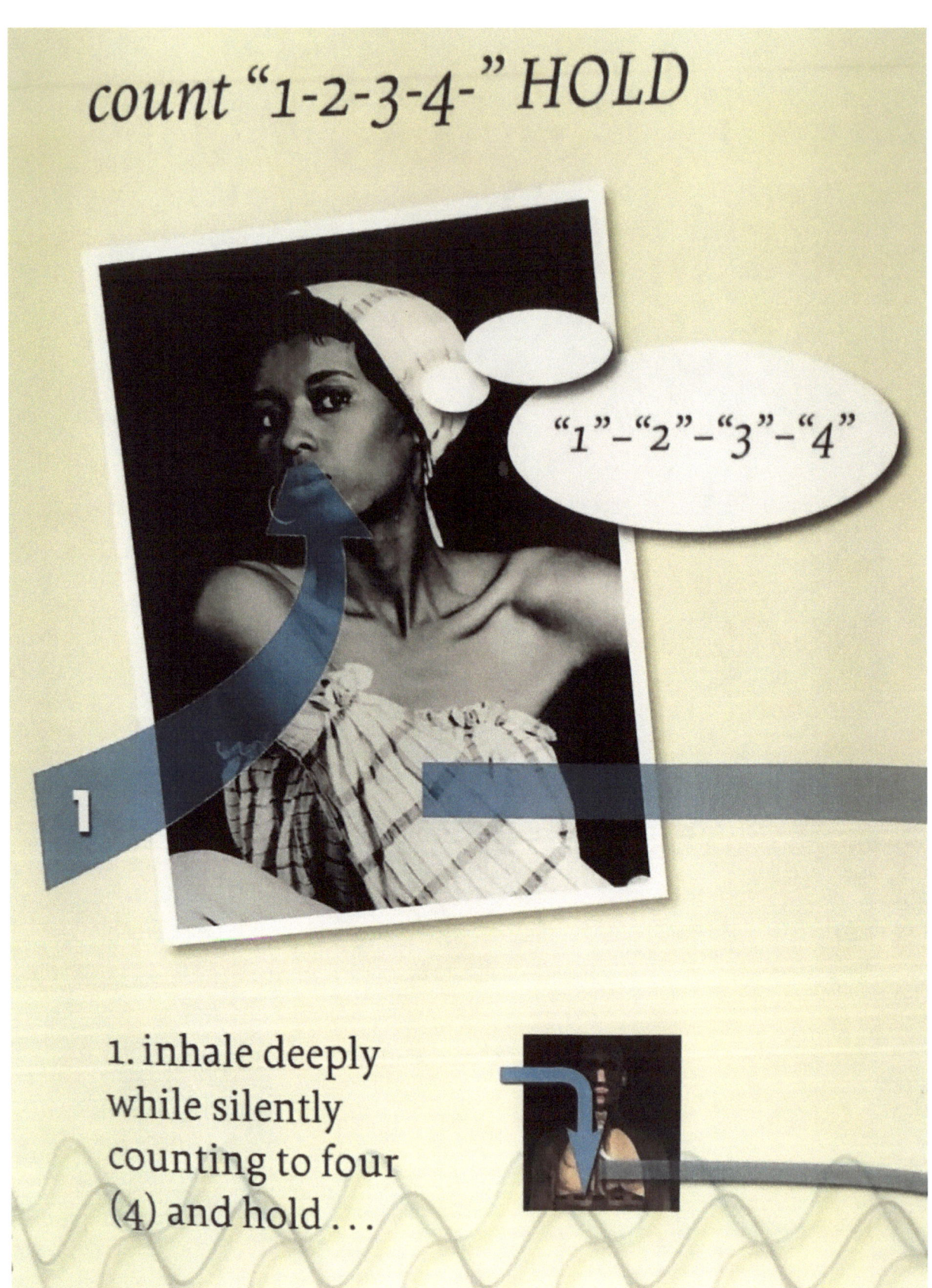

"1"-"2"-"3"-"4"

1. inhale deeply while silently counting to four (4) and hold...

count "-5-6-7..."

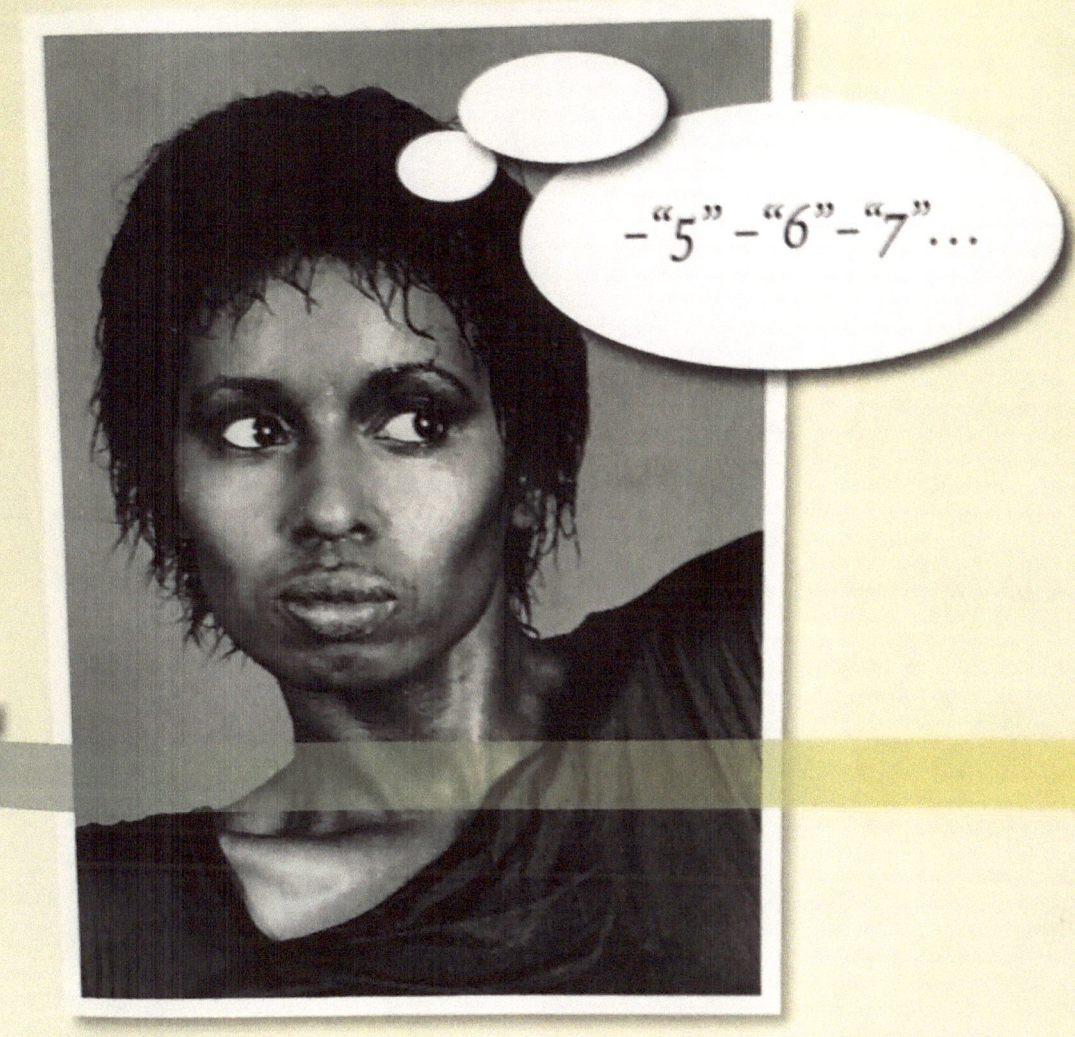

continue to hold while silently counting to eight (8)...

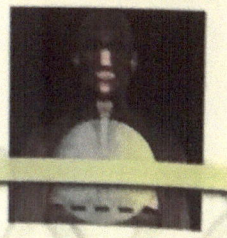

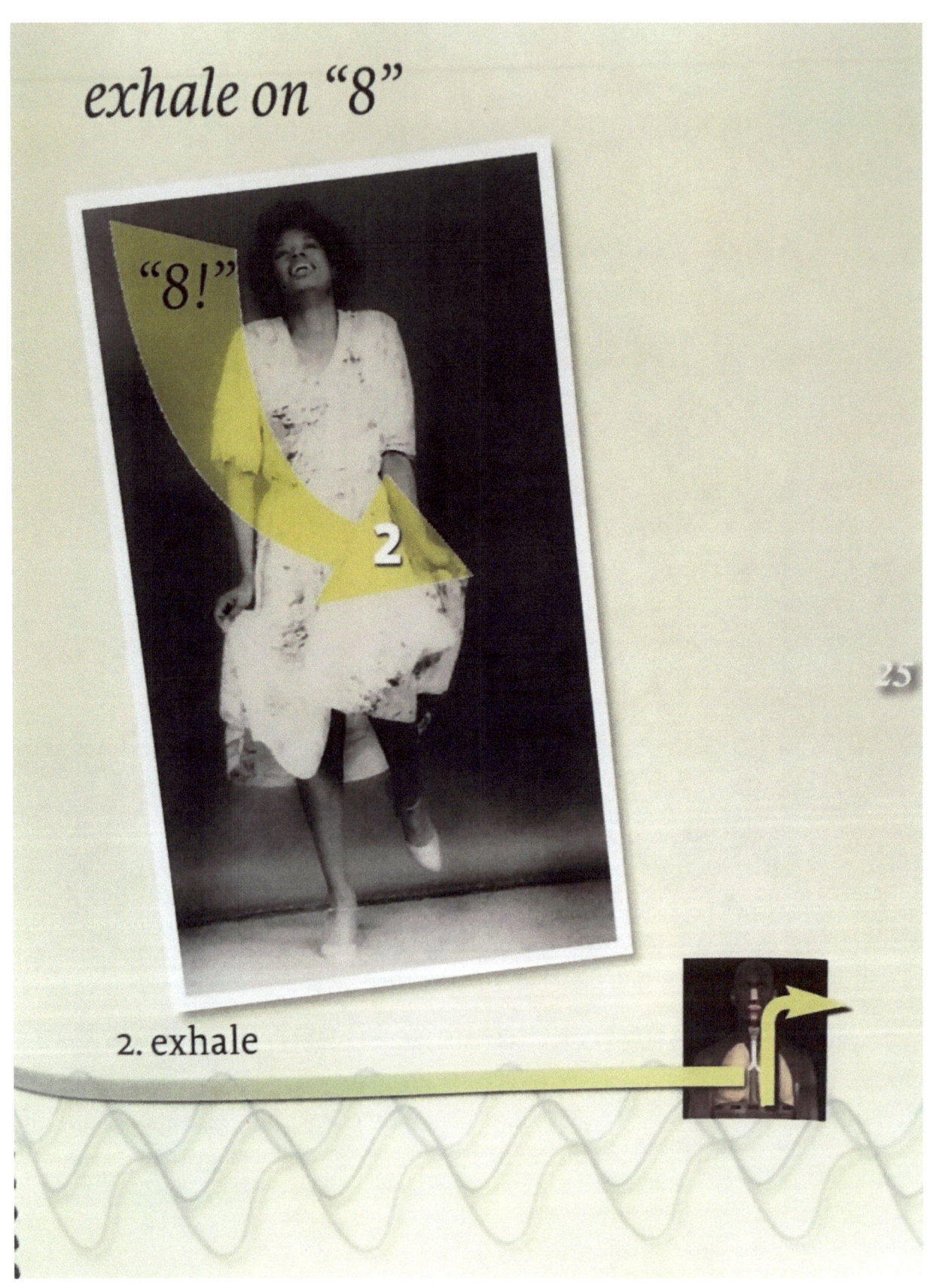

Movement

It's Universal! Most people love to dance! As we aged the white matter in our brain declined and movement such as dancing regularly can help maintain and improve brain health.

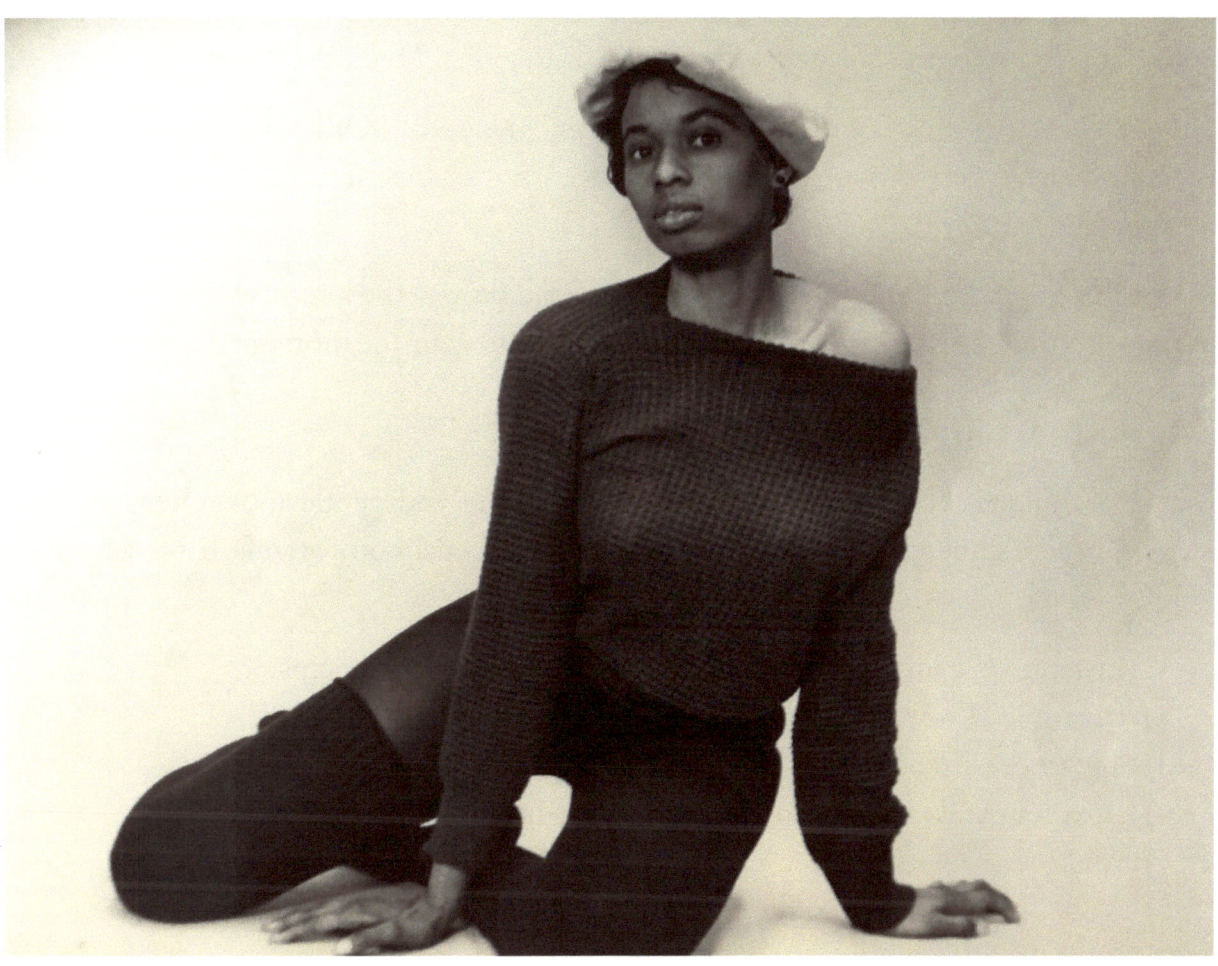

Research shows movement can improve mental health by boosting overall happiness. It's a low-impact, cardiopulmonary form of exercise that increases stamina, strengthens bones and muscles and staves off illness.

The New England Journal of Medicine published findings that stretching and movement on a regular basis is linked with a 76 percent reduction in dementia risk, whereas other physical activities such as bicycling, walking and performing housework were not associated with any decreased risk.

The study concluded that participation in leisure activities is associated with a reduced risk of dementia, even after adjusting for base-line cognitive status and after excluding of subjects with possible preclinical dementia.

Dancing was the only physical activity associated with a lower risk of dementia. Fewer than 10 subjects played golf or tennis, so the relation between these activities and dementia was not assessed.

Any physical activity increases neurotransmitters in the brain, which helps with depression, but it doesn't slow down diseases such as Alzheimer's, said Dr. Munawar Paracha, a neurologist affiliated with Kingman Regional Medical Center.

"Exercise always helps with mild depression," he said. "Other than that, physical activity doesn't slow down Alzheimer's. It does not change the course or progression of the disease."

Any form of physical exercise helps increase blood flow to the brain, which can improve symptoms of depression and make a person feel better for the moment, the doctor said.

Movement and Breathing Techniques

These techniques consist of breath work, stretching and gentle movement. First go through the technique without music and once you feel comfortable try it with your favorite song.

1) Listen to the initial couple of beat and once the music begins….
2) Breath in slowly and deeply…Exhale slowly and deeply (REPEAT)
3) Try to breath in sync with the beats of the music
4) Breath in and raised both arms over your head as you breath in
5) And lower them as you breathe out (REPEAT AGAIN).
6) Now lift your right shoulders 4 times and your left shoulder 4 times
7) Now lift both shoulders eight times.
8) Listen to the music for approximately 10 seconds.
9) Now put both hands on your abdomen and breath in and out

Repeat #4 only this time when you exhale continue to push all the air out as you lowered your arms (this is additional exhalation) which helps with anxiety. Repeat Again.

10) Listen to the music rhythms and beats for approximately 5 seconds.
11) Next place hands on thighs...**lift your right foot 4 times, repeat on the left side and then lift both feet (e.g. ** heel(s) up and down).
12) Repeat #6

Relax and close your eyes. Visualize a place or location that you remember making you smile and having a good feeling on your mind, body and soul (e.g. beach). Make a fist with the hand you write with to capture these good feelings and now relax this fist. NOTE: Whenever you feel stressed…make a fist with your dominant hand to capture that good feeling and then release.

Do these techniques daily.

Note: For a sample music for Movement go to www.audreygriefexpressionist.com

Cognitive Process

Studies show how different types of practice allow dancers to achieve peak performance by blending cerebral and cognitive thought process with muscle memory and "proprioception" held in the cerebellum.

A 2013 study published in Psychological Science magazine found that dancers can improve the ability to do complex moves by walking through them slowly and encoding the movement through "marking," which alleviates the cognitive and physical aspects of dance.

In general, dancing helps with motor control, proprioception and coordination, said Dr. Chris Bowers, physical therapist at KRMC. He could not speak to the neurological benefits.

Proprioception, or the perception of movement and spatial orientation, is important to maintain balance, he said. Dancing also improves the vestibular system, or inner ear, also critical for balance.

"I think it's not only having your mind active, but it's a great form of exercise for the whole body and person," said Debera Daugherty, executive director of Kathryn Heidenreich Adult Center.

"Music releases endorphins and gives you a better sense of well-being. I think it's a great social activity. They see their friends and meet new people."

Most of the 40 to 50 seniors who show up for the weekly dances are in their 60s and older, Daugherty said. Some of them get up and sing or play an instrument, which is also beneficial for the brain.

Dance and Brain

Mr. Emmanuel Boakye, author for the article, *"You won't believe the benefits of dancing for your brain!"* asked the question, *"Is there something you can do to preserve your youth and keep your brain well-functioning at all seasons of life?"* Start dancing! And here is why… Read more: https://yen.com.gh/62125-3-amazing-benefits-of-dancing-brain-dance-way-youth-great-memory.html.

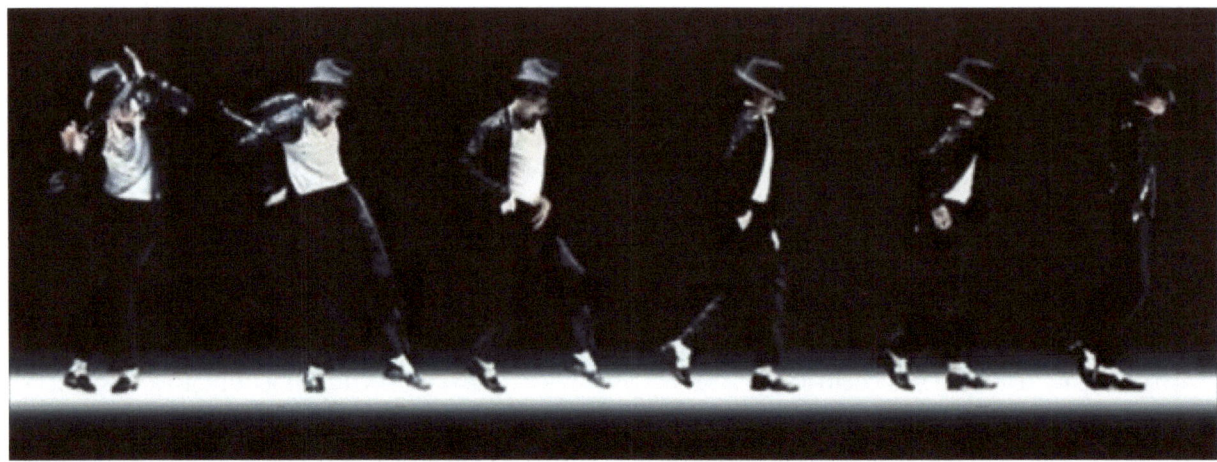

Scientists carried out numerous researches on how to help people resist aging and dementia. No one really wants to be out of their mind! They tried several physical activities, but some of them showed no result, such as cycling or swimming, for example. However, eventually, they discovered the thing that does the trick. Dancing keeps your brain young and hugely decreases the risk of dementia! Dancing can lower the possibility of dementia by 76%! Just compare this to 36% of reading impact, 47% of doing puzzles and 0% of playing golf. There is only one demand to meet to attain such a positive effect – you must dance and dance often! Read more: https://yen.com.gh/62125-3-amazing-benefits-of-dancing-brain-dance-way-youth-great-memory.html

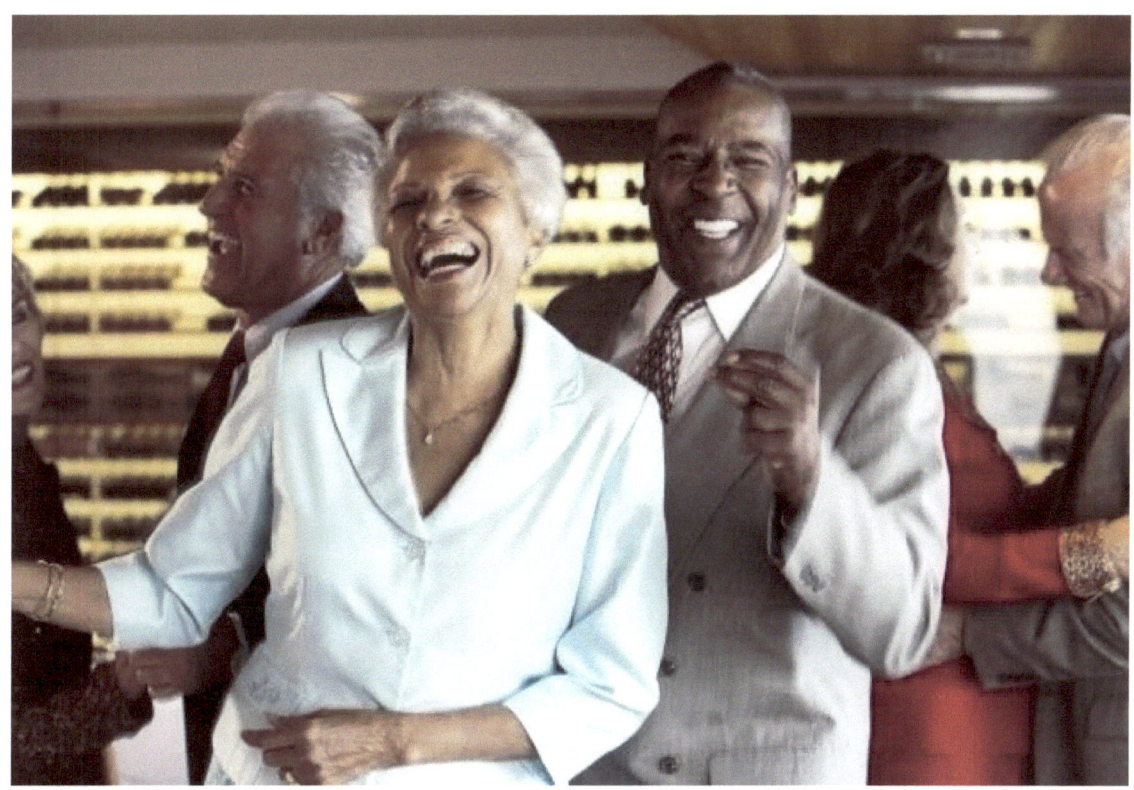

Here is what Dr. Robert Katzman has to say about it: "People who dance regularly have greater cognitive reserves and an increased complexity of neuronal synapses."

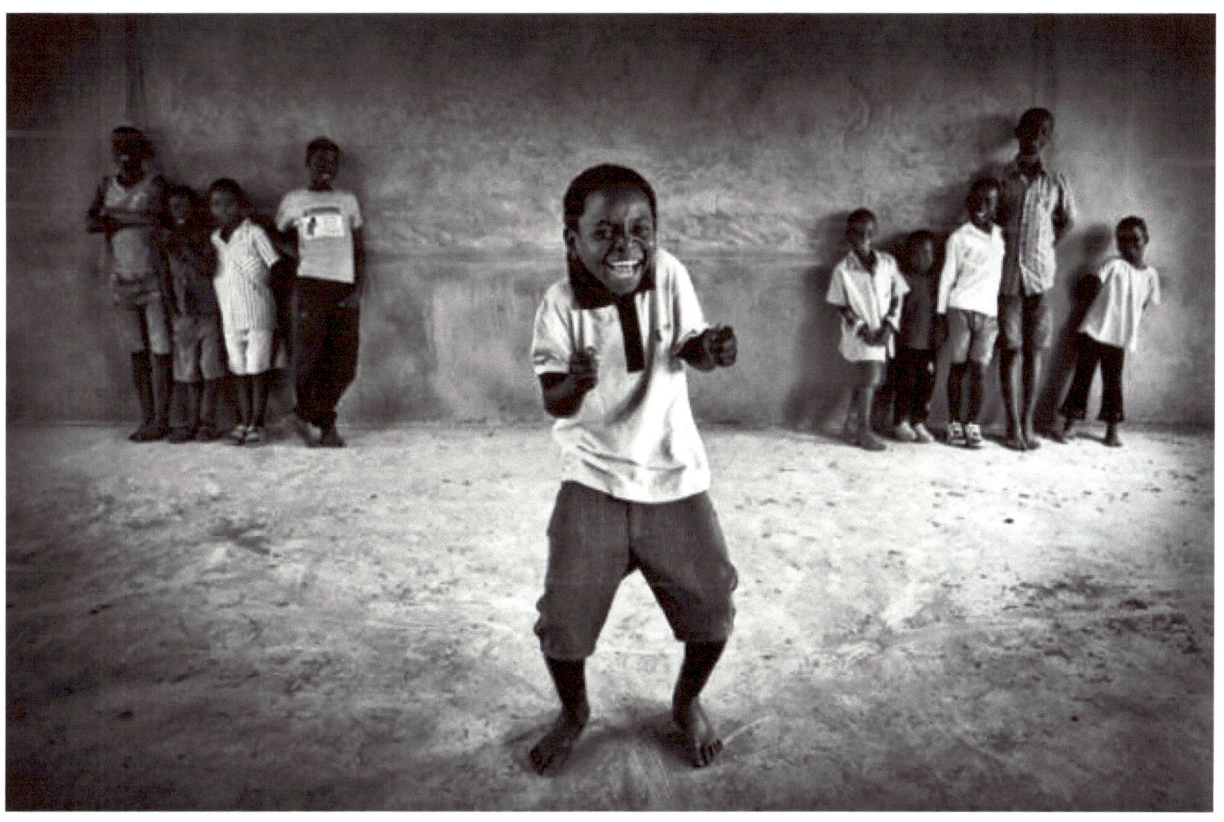

Dancing is the key to strengthening muscles with repeat repetition and our brain creates a memory or movement. The author also states, *"When you slowly repeat the movements repeatedly, you train your muscles to react without having to receive the brain signal each time. This way you bind your physical and cognitive abilities into one."*

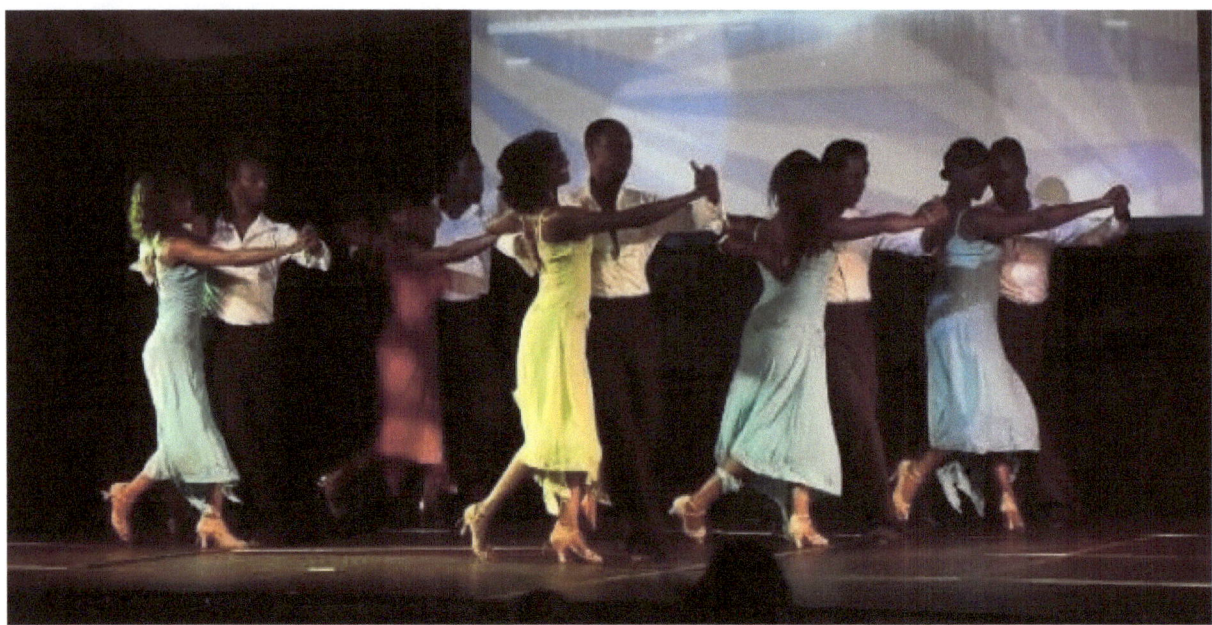

The author concluded, "Dancing creates new neural paths in the brain. It keeps your brain young and functional. When brain cells die, it becomes weaker, but when you dance the new cells start regenerating much faster. By dancing, you keep your memory sharp and prevent forgetting things. As you see, scientists have discovered a fun way to stay healthy and prevent dementia. Party to your heart's content and keep your brain going with these benefits of dancing!" Read more: https://yen.com.gh/62125-3-amazing-benefits-of-dancing-brain-dance-way-youth-great-memory.html

The Telomere Effect

As I was writing a conclusion to my book, I came across a TV program NHK World Japan, *"Today's Close-up."* The host Mr. Shinkhi Taketa states, "Will longing to stay healthy forever finally become a reality."

As physicians we learned in medical school that every cell in our body contain a human chromosome.

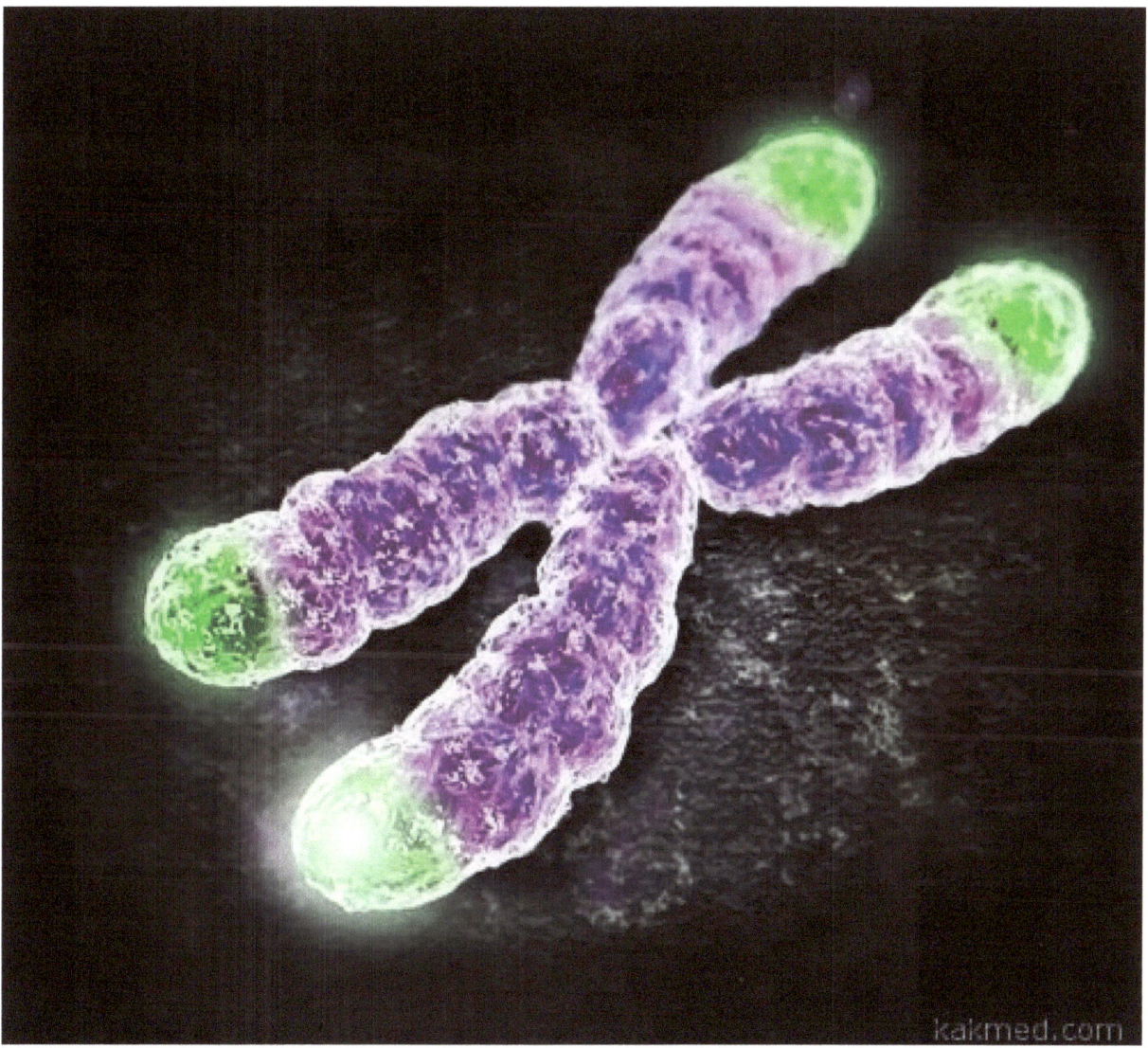

At the end of each chromosome is a region called a Telomere that holds the key to longevity and health. Each time a cell divides the telomere gets shorter. This phenomenon is believed to be involved in the aging process. Scientist are trying to make telomeres longer and prevent cancer and other illnesses. Ms. Elizabeth Blackburn, Nobel Laureate in Physiology or Medicine, and who's the author of the book, *"The*

Telomere Effect," states, *"We want people to understand they have some control over the lengthening of their telomeres." "There are certain things you can do that are not hard", Exercise, Diet, Sleep 7 or more hours and Relationships.* When the telomeres don't divide because they are too short a person is less healthy and looks older than their true age.

The latest studies addressed the questions, why do we age? How can we stay young? Biological studies have been increasingly focussed on the telomere effect. The book, *"The Telomere Effect,"* have captured wide world attention written by Elizabeth Blackburn who reached the conclusion that it is possible to prolong our health. She states, *"How well our arterioles are maintained is one of the things that is important for us to have a long health span."*

What caused shorten telomeres? New studies in the U.S. has found a factor that sped up the rate by which telomeres diminished. Namely, Psychological stress. Researcher Dr. Elissa Epel, studied the telomeres of the women who care for members of their family. The longer time they spent caregiving, the shorter and fewer their telomeres. Dr. Epel states that people with especially short telomeres have something in common. They worry a lot and are highly stress. They expect bad things to happen to them. These people are prone to cancer, cardiovascular disease and dementia. The shorter the telomeres the more the brain shrink and are a higher risk for less brain power.

Dr. Epel states, "There were certain findings that surprised me, such as meditation, love and relationships that works on a cellular level and have a positive impact on telomeres".

What Methods Could Increase Telomeres? Meditation Yoga

Instructions:

1) Breath in through your nostrils for 4 seconds – 4 times
2) Breath out through your mouth with purse lips for 4 seconds – 4 times
3) Thumb-to-Finger-Taps

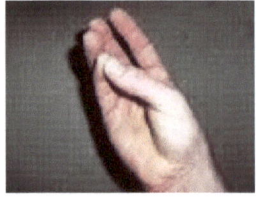

   a. Tap little finger to thumb with the tap say "SHAH"

b. Tap ring finger to thumb and with the tap say "TAH"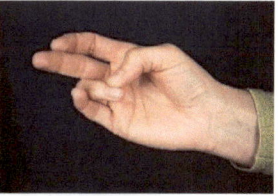

c. Tap middle finger to thumb and say" MAH"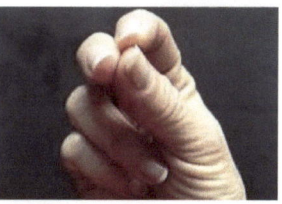

d. Tap index finger to thumb and say "YAH"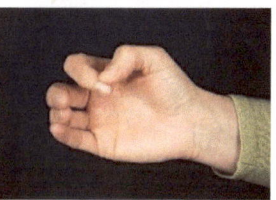

Method 1 - The Mantra

Repeat the Mantra, "SHAH, TAH, MAH and YAH out loud while you tap each finger with both hands. Start with 1 minute daily and work up to 10 minutes. Don't forget to do the breathing exercises prior to repeating the mantra. Now in your mind's eye focus on a shiny light and repeat the mantra over and over for 10 minutes.

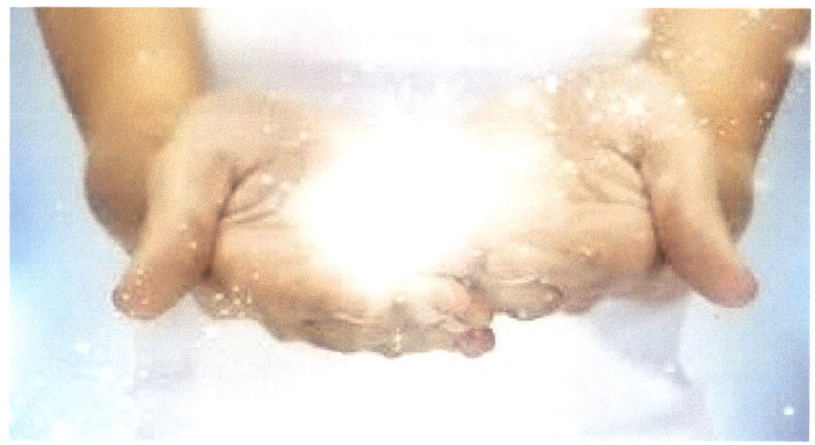

The Meditation Yoga Research

The research of 100 women over the age of 40 did this meditation yoga 12 minutes for two months and after testing showed their telomeres was increased via telomerase by 43%.

Practice

The Power is in the Hands

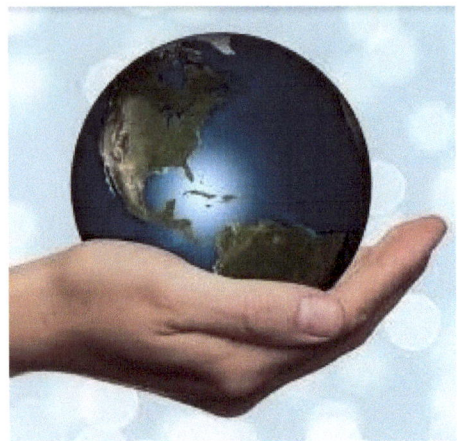

Observe the finger-to-tap illustrated in the following pictures.

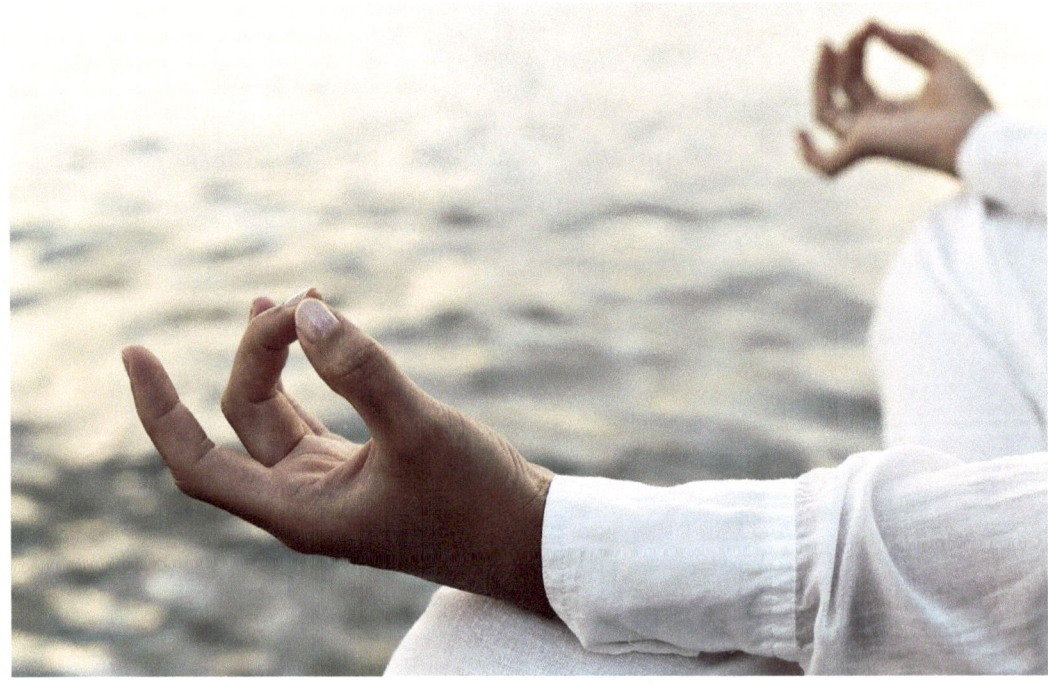

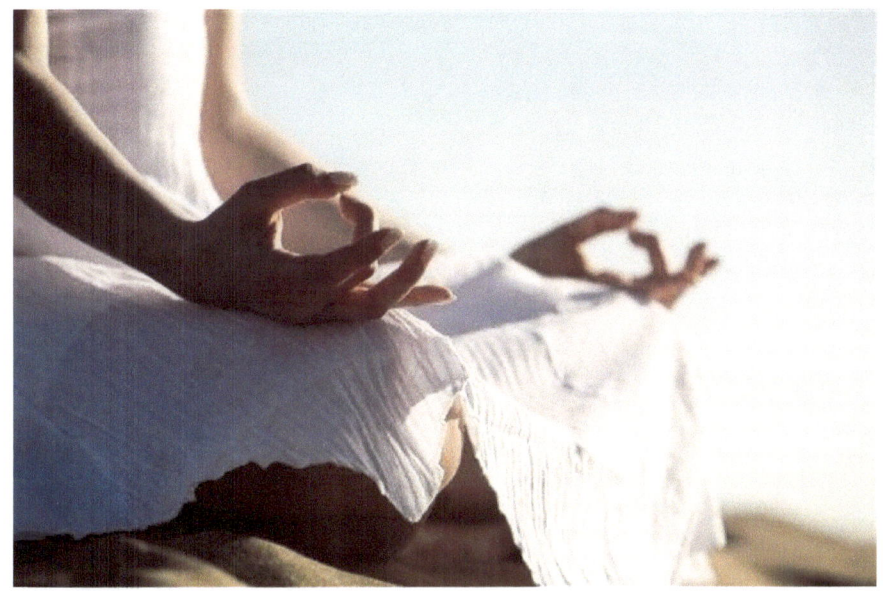
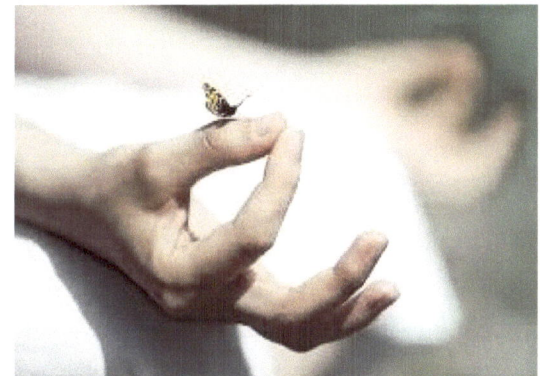
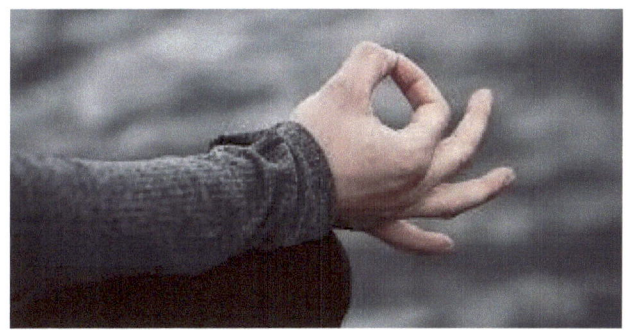
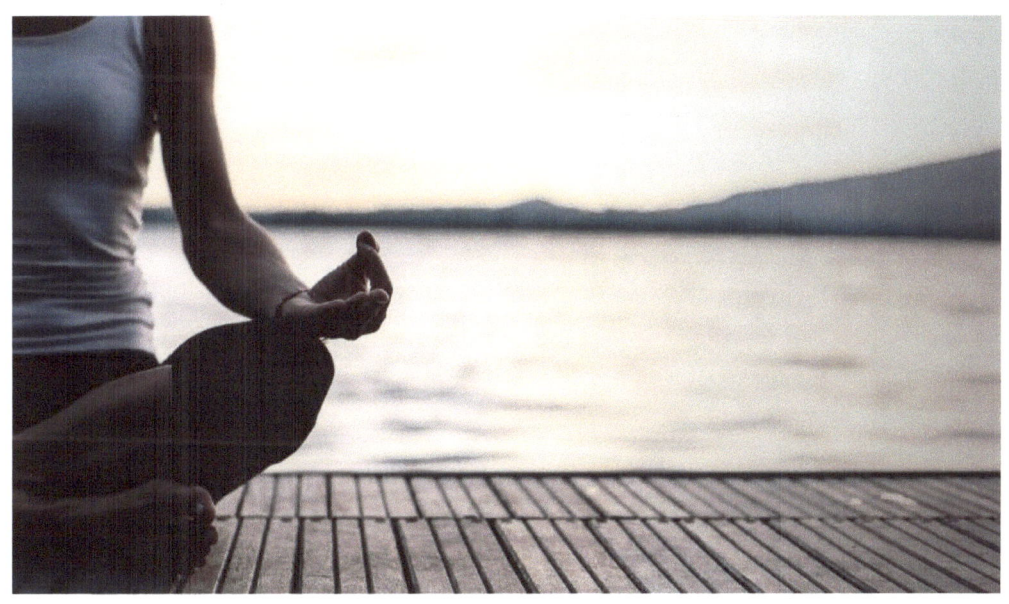

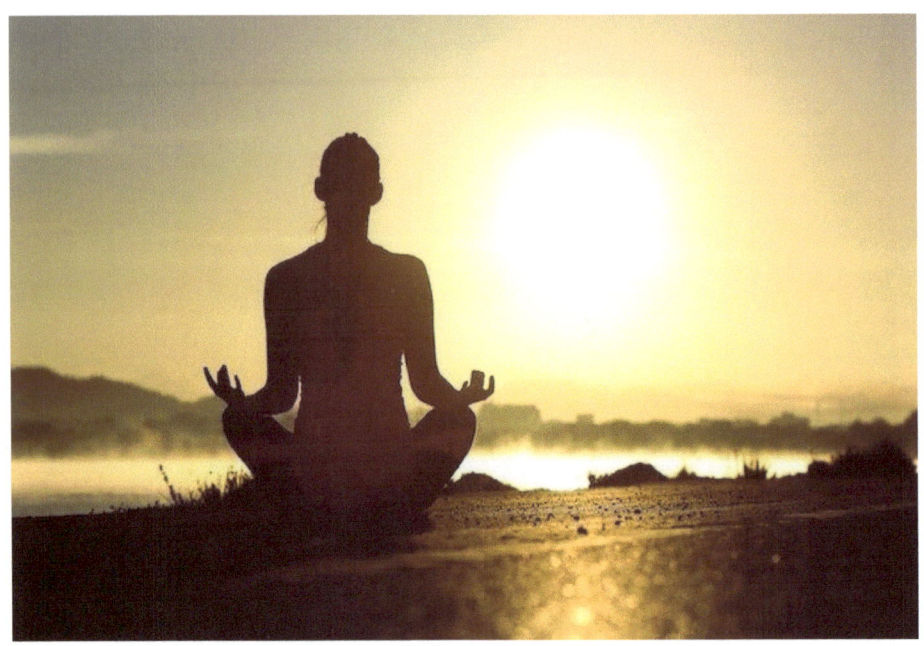

Method 2 – Enhancing Telomerase

Love and Intimacy

When we are in love it is an exhilarating experience and this emotion releases the good hormones in our brains, and we see the world more positive when we find that special person. The feeling of love affects our mental and physical well-being, and it have a direct impact on a cellular level.

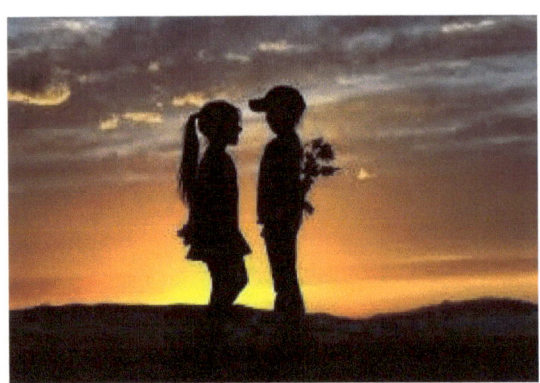
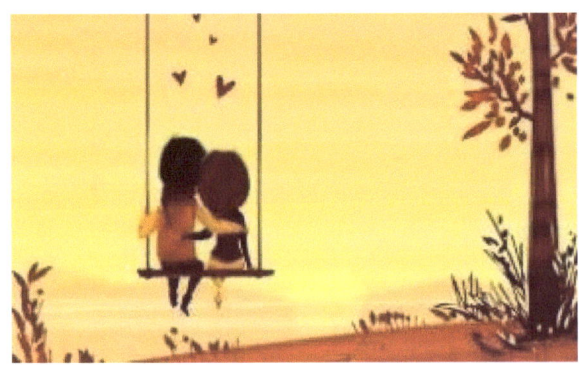

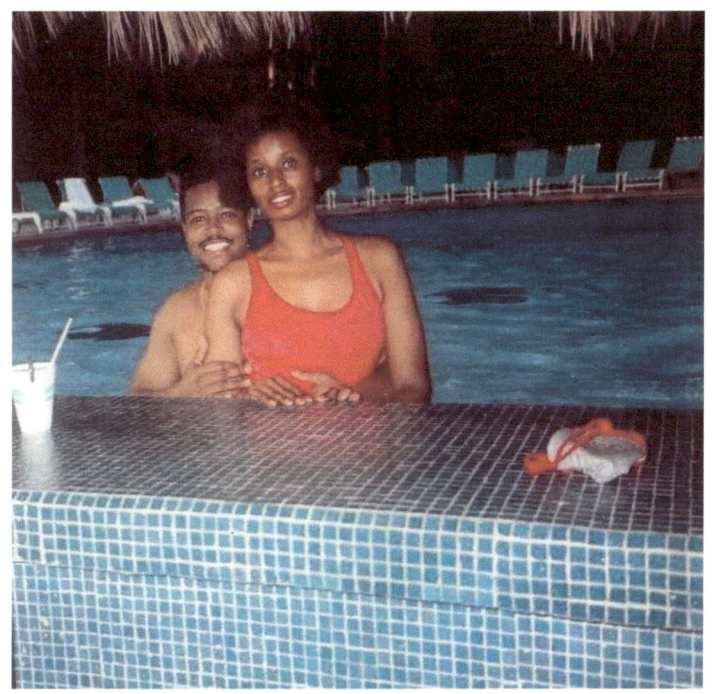

Method 3 – Friendship and Social Activities

Mr. Yoshiki Ishikawa, Public Health Researcher says, "It's really interesting one of the significant studies in the 21st century for preventive medicine is that being alone is as harmful as smoking." "The more stable a relationship people have and who are socially active can have an impact on a cellular level and activate the telomerase enzyme to extend one's telomeres which is a key to slowing aging and living a long and healthy life.

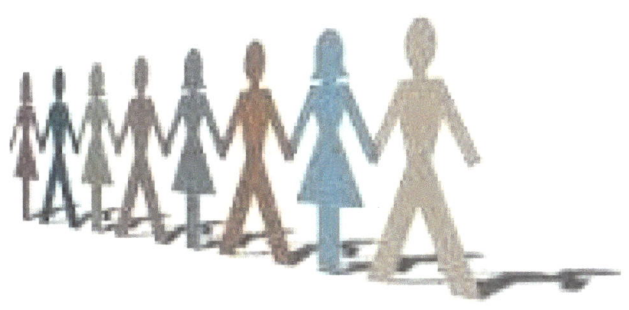

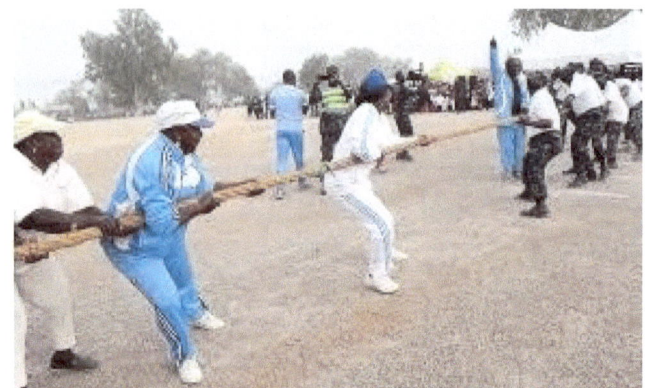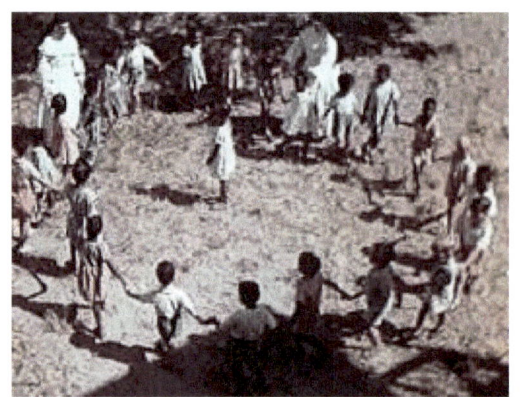

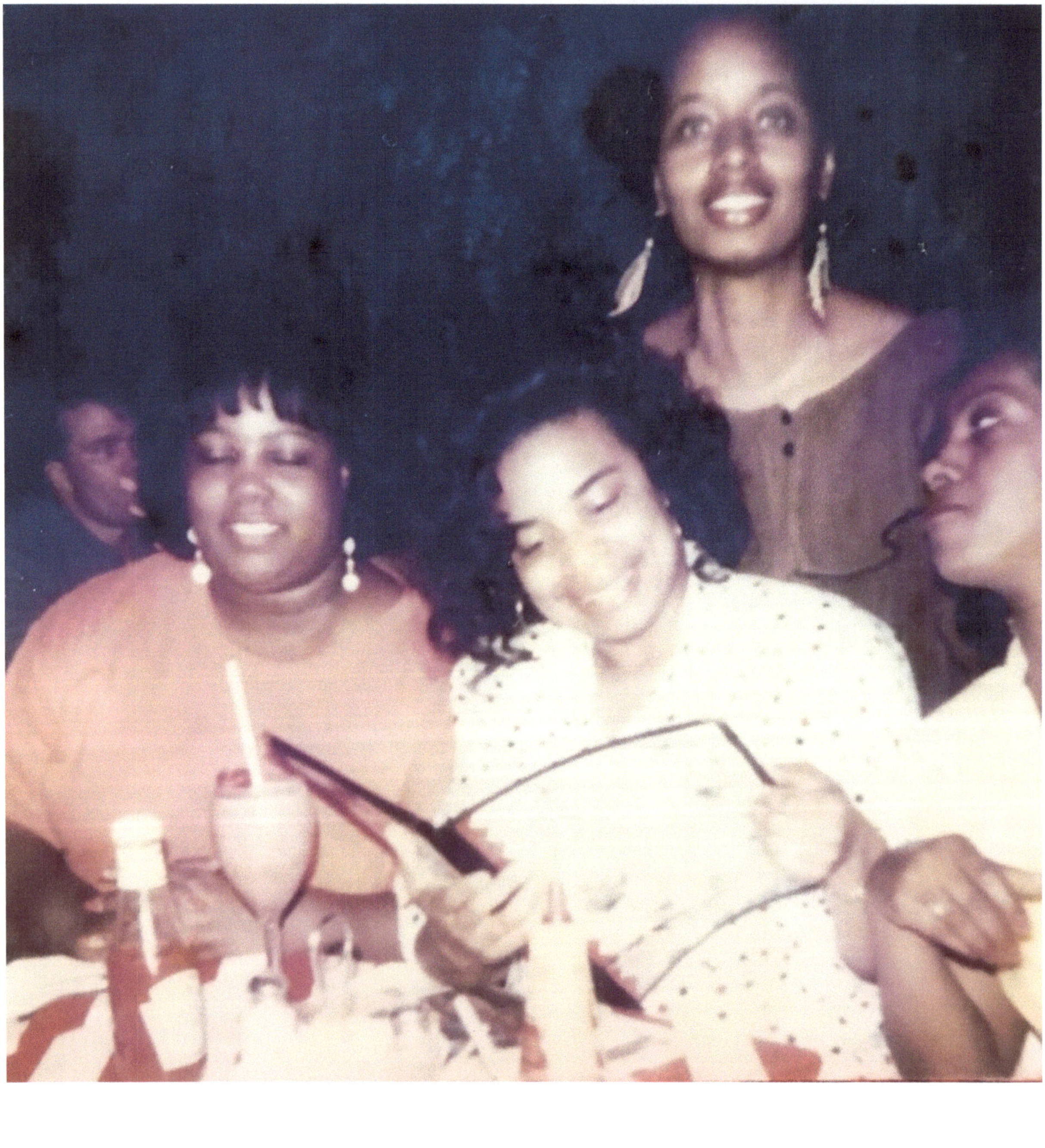

Method 4 – Nature and You

Studies have shown if you take daily walks and take notice of nature and her greenery it will relax the total body and bring a harmonious balance and peace of mind.

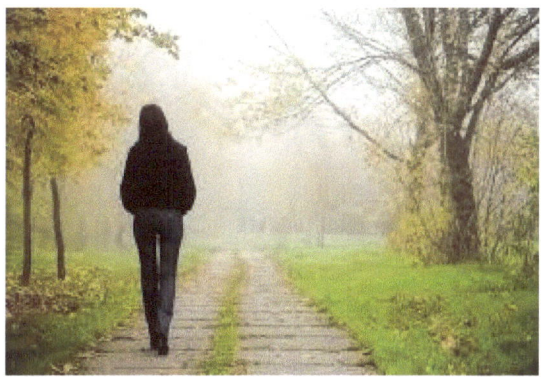

Also, if you walk with someone who you care for is an added bonus of mental and physical well-being

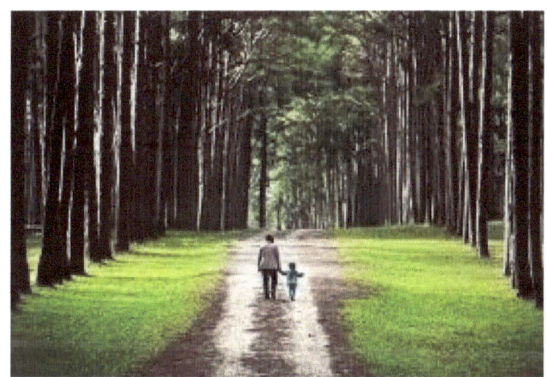

Dr. Dean Ornish, President, Preventive Medicine Research Institute is also studying telomerase role in extending longevity. His study was done on a group of cancer patients which included a 4 part regimen.

1) Meditation

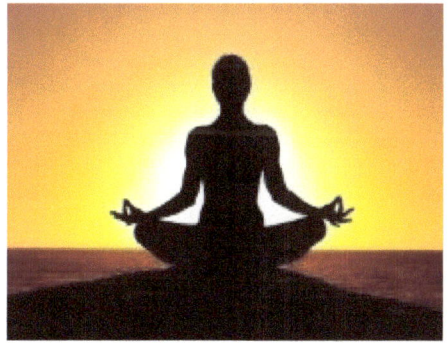

2) Aerobic Exercise

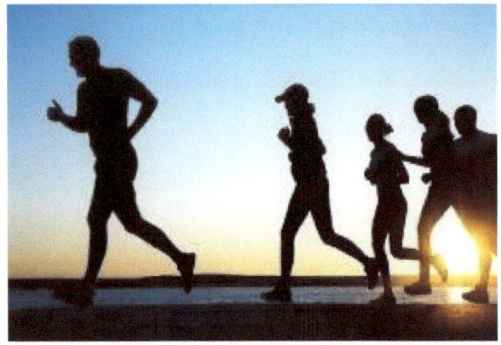

3) Walking daily for 30 minutes

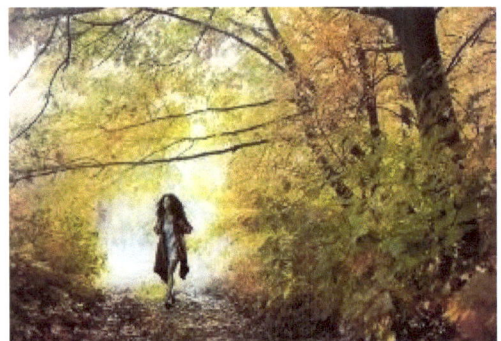

4) Vegetable based diet

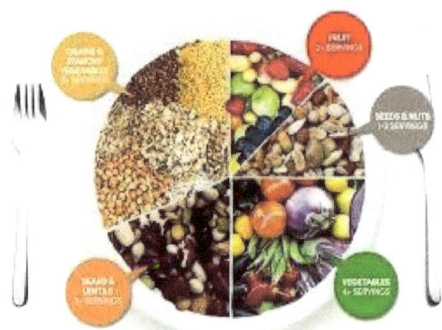

Lastly, they were offered counseling sessions once a week. The goal was for them to learn the importance of interpersonal relationships, such as, those with their families and neighbors. Dr. Ornish states, *"What we call social support which is really love and intimacy."* *"Study after study have shown that people who are lonely and depressed are treated more and likely to be sick and die prematurely for pretty much every cause; as well as have shorter telomeres."* After continuing the program for 5 years the subjects saw their telomeres grow by an average of 10%, and the spread of their cancer also slowed. Dr. Dean states, "Simple changes can make such a powerful difference." "In effect, begin to reverse aging on a cellular level.

How does this work?

Dr. Helen Lavretsky, a researcher and psychiatrist states, when we are stressed the parasympathetic system vagal response is reduced, and the sympathetic or stress hormones goes up. The methods for extending telomerase, such as, meditation, visualization, imagination, exercise and increased green vegetables equalizes and rebalance both the parasympathetic and sympathetic system. They come together and activate the telomerase to extend the telomeres. It all begins at the DNA. The new cells divide and replicate the lengthening of the telomeres.

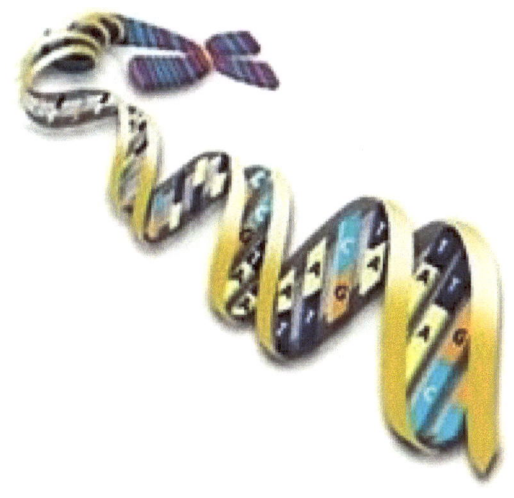

Reflection

What is the reflection of your life? Is it in balance with mind, body and spirit?

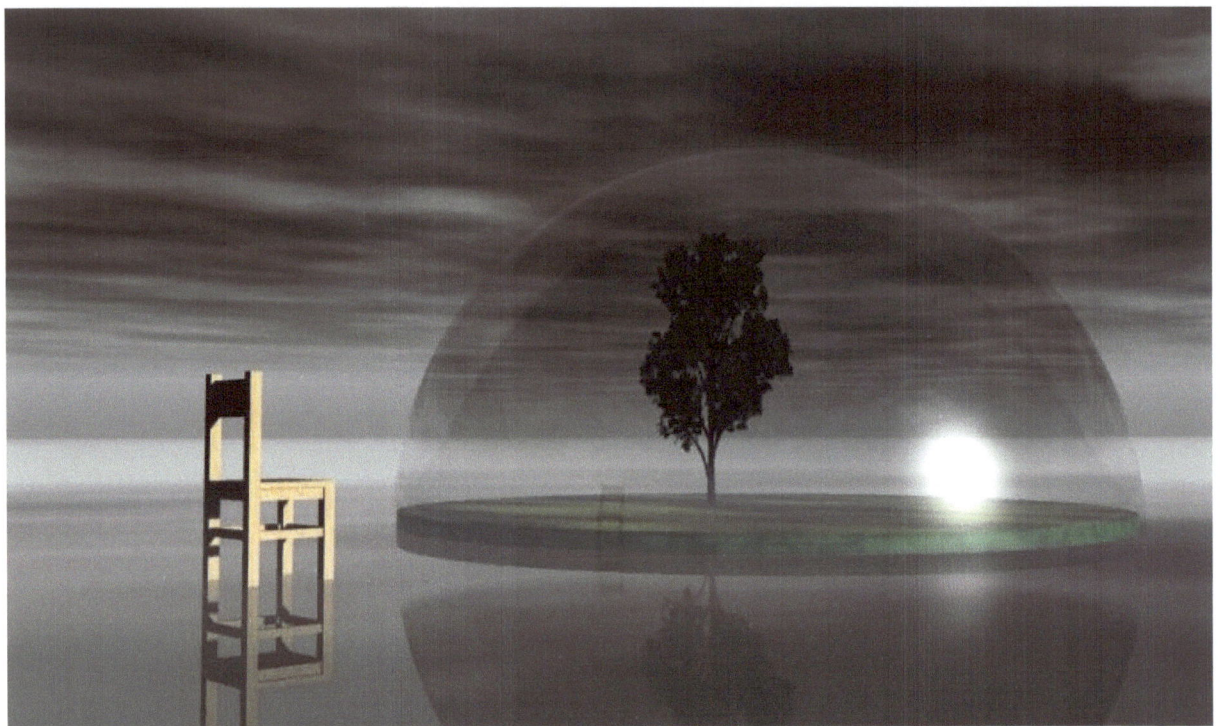

The creative tools in this book should have helped you answer these questions. What is missing in your life? Is your chair empty? Seeing your goals and dreams from afar with the sunset disappearing and so are your opportunities. The empty chair is metonym *for a position of power and influence, so empty chair is easily turned into a metonym of abdicated power or influence. Therefore, the chair is an opportunity for you to succeed in life, but fear is keeping you from sitting and gaining the power and influence waiting for you.*

The Umbrella Story

Do you ever walk outside, and the weather is cloudy and rainy? The weather can affect our mood. If the sun is out it brightens our mood. If it's cloudy our mood is gloomy. The umbrella story is that we determine our mood whether it's sunny or cloudy. This is because we must establish a higher level of thinking which is a positive state of mind, and not depend on what it look like outside to determine it. The Power is within you to retrain the brain to think a certain way. What you want is to shift to the left prefrontal cortex (The Einstein or Genius part of the brain) from the right prefrontal cortex (Frankenstein part of the brain). The latest scientific findings establish that you can change your life by changing your brain. For many years, scientist believed that your brain was a static, hard-wired organ, but the study of Neuroplasticity has proven otherwise. Your brain is forming new connections and growing new brain cells every day. A study published in clinical psychology review suggest that, when you practice a variety of specific brain correlated activities you can transform your health, finances, career and relationship.

Your World is Upside Down

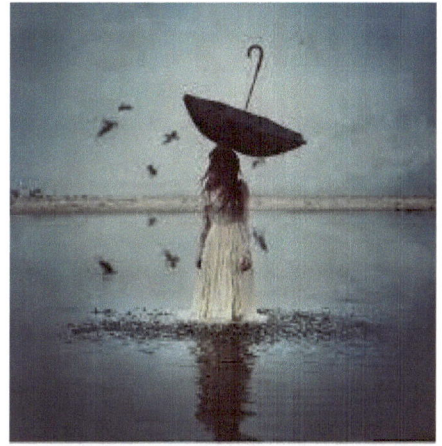

Your World is Cloudy

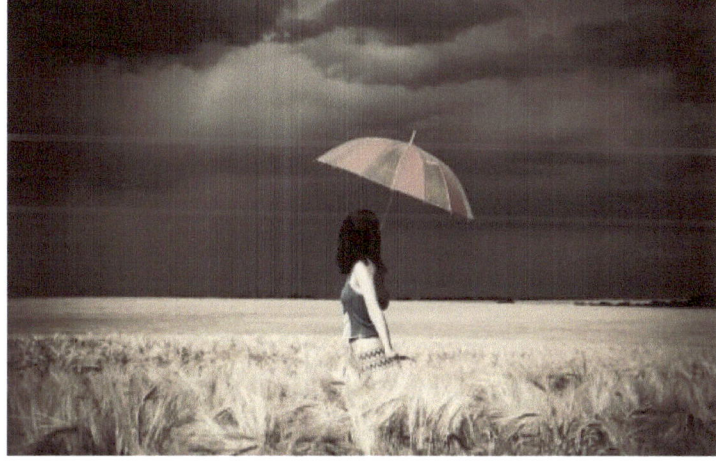

Your World is Full of Sunshine

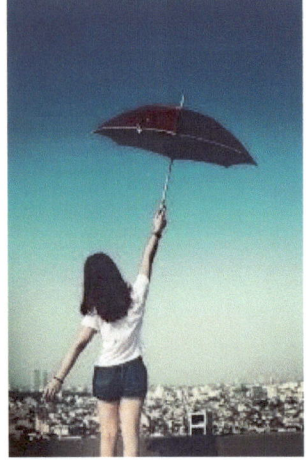

A Reflection of a Balanced Life

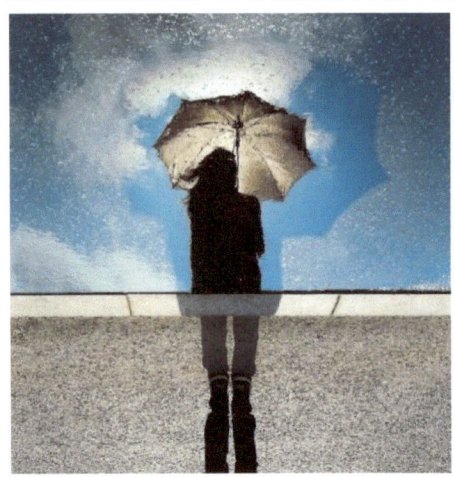

A World of Peace, Happiness and Joy

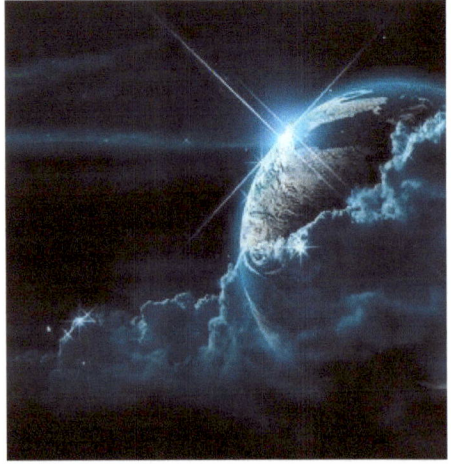

Spirituality and the Grief Connection

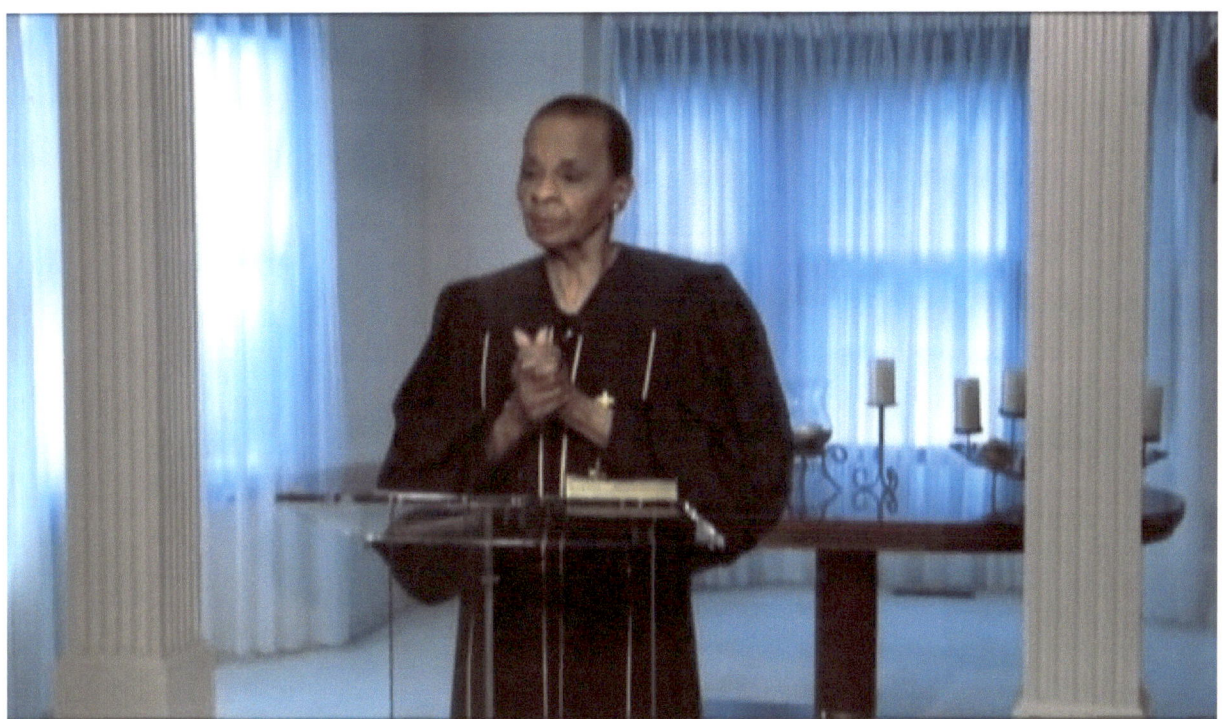

The Grief Connection

I am initiating this discussion with the premise that there is a proper alignment between mind, body and spirit; when this alignment is disturbed it results in disharmony and mental illness.

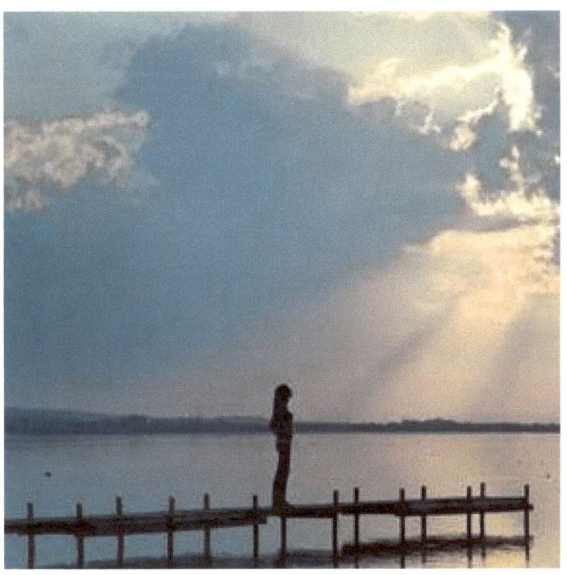

I was indoctrinated, in my youth with the religious belief that there was a God who created the universe; and fashioned a tri-part being in his own image. He called his creation a man, and gave him a body, a soul and spirit. The **Body** is the vessel which functions to transport man's soul and spirit through time on an earthly journey to meet his or her destiny. The **Soul** is the very essence of man's being. It is his mind, his will, and his emotion. The **Spirit** is that part of us that allows us to communicate with God. Religion teaches us that God gave man and woman a free will and time honored "principles of living" on which to exercise this free will. The religious person believes that if a man or woman lives according to these basic biblical principles, his or her spiritual life will be whole; his earthly journey fruitful, and his salvation assured. On the other hand, if a man or woman chooses not to live by these principles their spiritual life will be empty, his or her earthy journey rocky and they will have no opportunity for salvation. Is there a relationship between religion, spirituality, depression and grief? Wikipedia says, "Historically, the words religious and spiritual have been used synonymously to describe all the various aspects of the concept of religion, but in contemporary usage spirituality has often been associated with the interior life of the individual, placing an emphasis upon well-being of the "mind-body-spirit, while religion refers to organization or communal dimension."

What about people who are not spiritual or who do not believe in God? Do these principles apply to them? Yes, these basic principles even apply to those who are not spiritual or who claim not to believe in God. The Apostle Paul stated that God equipped man with a conscious to guide him on his earthly journey regarding right and wrong **(II Corinthians 4:1-7).**

Religion or Spirituality are very personal and very hard to define. They mean different things to different people. Some have said that God created man with a space that only he can fill; and that our time on earth is an intense personal search for something to fill that space which God has created in us. It has been said that if man can't find God, he will create one. This belief is supported by Old Testament scripture **(Exodus 32:1-5),** citing that even the Israelites, God's chosen people grew impatience waiting for Moses to return from conferencing with the living God and they pleaded with Aaron to make them an idol God so that they could have something concrete to worship. Thus, Aaron obliged them by creating a Golden Calf.

Dr. Avid Steere book, Spiritual Presence in Psychotherapy, describes spiritual homelessness. The spiritually homeless are those whose quest for meaning and wholeness has carried them away from their church home. They wander the streets in search of a place to house their thirst for healing and inner peace. They have a "consumer mentality," which demands services they no longer find viable or satisfying in organized religious life. Those who are spiritually homeless seek two things. The first is spiritual direction that can bring meaning or purpose to their lives, a certain sense of inner fulfillment or satisfying devotion to something sacred. The second is healing, not simply physical and emotional healing, but wholeness and well-being that comes from facing one's vicissitudes, coping with the estrangement that can overwhelm their personal relationships as couples, families, friends, or coworkers. This concern for wholeness which the root meaning of the word "holy," is the driving force behind spiritual homelessness, which, in turn provides the background for a rapprochement between the field of psychiatry and spirituality.

There is a thin line between normal and abnormal behavior; between psychiatric illness and somatic illness. We are all plagued by personal demons. These demons may on occasion cause a malalignment of our mind body spirit axis, resulting in psychiatric stress or illness. We use different techniques to realign ourselves to a more harmonious relationship of self.

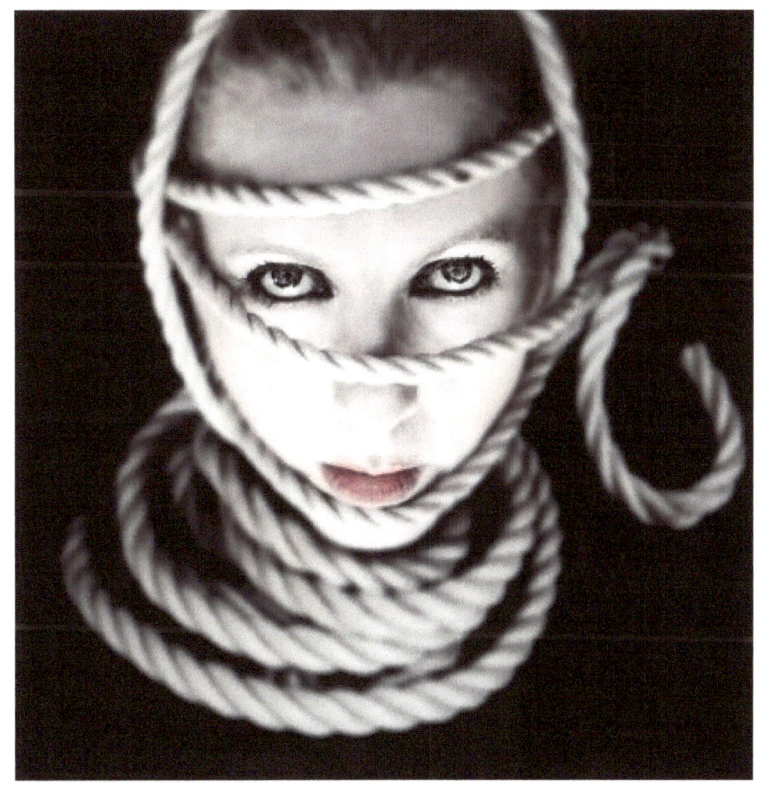

Case in point, **Ms. CB,** is a 37-year-old psychiatrically disabled Puerto Rican woman, *a Fundamentalist Christian,* who was admitted for exhibiting symptoms of auditory and visual hallucinations; bizarre persecutory delusion of a demonic theme and paranoia. She would verbalize over and over in **Spanish, *"el diablo tiene cuerdas alrededor de mi cabeza* or English translation, "the devil has ropes around my head." Ms. CB** proceeded to scream, "el *diablo puso polvo blanco en mi cara;"* or the devil put white powder on my face*.*

Ms. CB, proceeded to scream, "I don't believe in doctors"; "the devil sends the doctors"; and the "spirits think I am crazy!"

My diverse background and cultures provided me the tools to understand ***Ms. CB's*** frame of reference at the time of her admission. I was able to **connect** with her through language and culture. She exhibited psychopathological distortion of normative religious beliefs which can be seen in schizophrenic patients, some of whom believe, during the prodromal/early stages of their illness, that special powers have been given to them by divine sources and they can use these powers to influence other people's actions or the outcome of events affecting their families, friends and communities. ***Ms. CB's*** psychosis were more florid, with the belief that she was possessed by some other worldly force (e.g. the spirit of an ancestor or deity, a malevolent spirit such as the devil); in psychiatry, possession is by an alternative personality, as in the dissociative fragmentation of personality. ***Ms. CB*** also had feelings of guilt because she's a ***Christian*** and was ***"living in sin"*** with her boyfriend of 10 years. She said**, God's eye was watching her from heaven.**

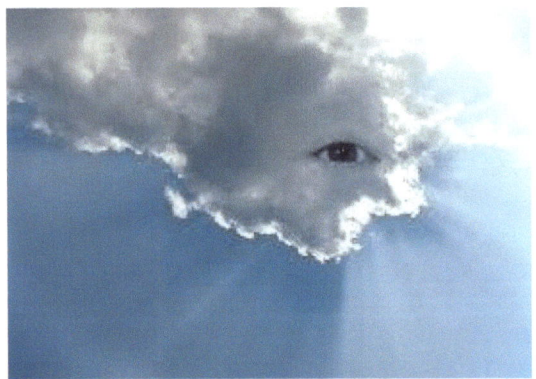

According to Dr. Glen Gabbard a psychoanalyst, he believed that when working with patients with a religious fixation, psychosis, and fragile egos, therapeutic alliance is more difficult to develop and maintain. This proved to be true working with ***Ms. CB,*** was both a rewarding and challenging patient. Treating ***Ms. CB,*** provided a multifaceted of treatment choices. She was suffering from paranoid schizophrenia with disturbances in the areas of thoughts, feelings, perceptions, behaviors, and cognition. ***Ms. CB,*** was plagued with troublesome thoughts. For example, delusional themes of persecution and obsessional thinking about the "devil." ***Ms. CB's*** feelings also proved disturbing. She was easily irritable and physically assaulted her property manager. Disruptive perception, such as auditory and visual hallucinations. ***Ms. CB's*** cognitive capacities were altered as well. For example, she showed signs of confusion and poor concentration probably secondary to her psychosis. Finally, **Ms. CB's** evidenced problematic and upsetting behaviors, such as restlessness, and frequent fighting with common-in-law husband.

After two weeks of inpatient hospitalization and a structure day program, **Ms. CB** was seen on an outpatient basis. This would involve individual therapy with maintaining a long acting IM antipsychotic, creativity and change her old story to a new one. The creative component was difficult to figure out seeing **Ms. CB**, as an inpatient because her behavior was so violent and psychosis very prominent; the staff first goal was to stabilize her on the appropriate medication. To get a clearer understanding on what **Ms. CB** likes to do creatively I spoke with her partner who informed me that she likes romantic music, and her favorite artist is Luis Miguel. The Ah hah! moment came to me because 2 years prior I was living in Puerto Rico and Luis Miguel was one of my favorite artists and I had a lot of music. He also said that Ms. CB likes to read the bible daily, and her favorite scripture was Psalms 23rd. I had another Ah hah! Moment because when I was living in New York attending drama school I read Psalms 23 to relieve stress and build confidence.

Ms. CB was obese, with a history of hypertension and a new onset of type II diabetes. There was ongoing communication with her primary care physician to address her physical treatments. **Ms. CB** education about her illness was also an ongoing process. Once she was stabilized on her medications, the goal was to initially provide weekly individual supportive therapy. Studies have shown that the effect of individual psychotherapy in the treatment schizophrenia have been helpful and additive to the effects of pharmacological treatment. During these weekly sessions we focused on self and ego. These sessions were not at the level of Freud's structural theory and model of self as an intrapsychic representation. It involved **Ms. CB's** subjective experiences and interactions with the world. There was also an overlap with cognitive therapy. Dr. Judith Beck's book, ***Cognitive Therapy: Basics and Beyond,*** theorized that there was a thinking disorder at the core of the psychiatric syndromes such as depression and anxiety. This disorder was reflected in a systematic bias in the way the patients interpreted experiences. However, cognitive therapy has been used in schizophrenic patients to improve cognitive distortion, reduce distractibility and correct errors in judgment. **Ms. CB** was able to ameliorate some of her delusional beliefs by using this method. After one year of therapy, her mental life and behavior had evolved into a more positive form.

In the beginning of **Ms. CB** second year of therapy, we switched to the emphasis on self-healing, spiritual awakening, and prevention of relapses (e.g. continual compliance with her medications). I would provide **Ms. CB** Prolixin injections every 2 weeks, and she continued to do well with her compliance with weekly sessions. Her daily practiced of meditation would begin with simple breathing of inhalation and exhalation; listening to Luis Miguel music with her eyes and the visualization of herself in a positive situation; and to find peace with self, and environment-completed the balance. I would have **Ms. CB** bring her bible into the office and read Psalms 23rd to me. I asked Ms. CB to write down words that was important to her in this scripture. From this I pulled out Affirmations for **Ms. CB** to read out loud daily. The goal was to established focus, organization and discipline for **Ms. CB** Through repetition of speaking daily positive words would build confidence, courage, and a new pattern of thinking. This would also be her anchor in times of stress, fear and worry. The Psalms 23 would create a happy family atmosphere and a better understanding of her Christian experience and a positive relationship with God.

In fact, the very essence of religion is to adjust the mind and soul of a person. A mind which thinks in error or drastic negativity is a sick mind. **Ms. CB** and I was on a positive path together to change this pattern of thinking.

Psalms 23 – The Word

Each one of us can map his or her destiny through their **WORDS**. There is **POWER IN YOUR WORDS!** *If you change the way you see things, the things you see will change.*

THE LORD IS MY SHEPHERD – *That's Protection!*

I SHALL NOT WANT – *That's Supply!*

HE MAKETH ME TO LIE DOWN IN GREEN PASTURES – **That's Rest!**

HE LEADETH ME BESIDE THE STILL WATERS – **That Calmness!**

HE RESTORETH MY SOUL – **That's Healing!**

HE LEADETH ME IN THE PATHS OF RIGHTEOUSNESS –

FOR HIS NAME SAKE – **That's Guidance!**

YEA, THOUGH I WALK THROUGH THE VALLEY OF THE SHADOW OF DEATH – **That's Testing!**

I WILL FEAR NO EVIL – **That's Faith**

FOR THOU ART WITH ME, THE ROD AND THY STAFF THEY COMFORT ME – **That's Discipline!**

THOU PREPAREST A TABLE BEFORE ME IN THE PRESENCE OF MINE ENEMIES – **That's Hope!**

THOU ANOINTS MY HEAD WITH OIL – **That's Blessings!**

MY CUP RUNNETH OVER – **That's Abundance!**

SURELY, GOODNESS AND MERCY SHALL FOLLOW ME ALL THE DAYS OF MY LIFE – **That's Favor!**

AND I WILL DWELL IN THE HOUSE OF THE LORD FOREVER – **That's Security and Eternity! –** Amen

In collaboration, the patient and I agreed to the following schedule. She was to read it the first thing when she awakened in the morning. Read it carefully, meditatively, and prayerfully. Immediately after breakfast, she was to do the same thing. Also, immediately after lunch, again after dinner, and, finally, the last thing before she went to bed. It was not to be a quick, hurried reading. She was to think about each phrase, giving her mind time to soak up as much of the meaning as possible. The goal of the Psalms 23 daily affirmation was to established focus and discipline. Secondly to build up trust and Faith in God, to ensure that she wasn't being judged for "living in sin."

Initially, it was difficult for **Ms. CB** to maintain this schedule, but she was allowed flexibility to change it. She wanted to default back to old habits…the old story. We become what we think and feel. Our beliefs become our reality. The beliefs within us determine our perception of what surrounds us, including what and how we select, register and process. Change is difficult because the brain's preference is for energetic economy. The brain strives first to transform experience as quickly as possible to habit by building new neurons and networks as the default mode.

We began to write a new story through creativity, movement, imagination and visualization. Going through these new modalities with **Ms. CB** where awkward and uncomfortable while triggering feelings of doubt and anxiety. These are predictable reactions in the mind/brain to new stimuli, requiring a shift from the automatic mode into an active level of processing. Change creates discontinuity and disrupts the "normal" state of cohesion. Enough practice, however, firmly establishes new neural pathways and networks and results ultimately in the creative pattern done without much thought or physical effort.

The success with this client was three-folded: First **Ms. CB** was compliant with treatment and medications. Second, she found her own creativity and uniqueness in handling life's challenges. Thirdly, she took ownership of her story and begin to change old habits and write a new life story. Finally, the patient and I worked together in collaboration with her treatment, and she trust me as her physician.

Finally, we want healing in the broadest sense, not just of our emotional disorders. Therefore, we need to shift the paradigm and stopped putting psychiatric patients in a "box" but as human beings with their own uniqueness who can contribute to themselves and the larger society as functioning person.

When grieving, you may experience intense emotions, find yourselves disoriented and unable to concentrate, or see that you are not behaving as you usually do. You may feel physically ill, experiencing a variety of aches and pains. And grief can also can affect your sense of spirituality.

Whatever your spirituality, losses can really test those beliefs. One of the issues in grief is to reconnect, maybe even rebuild, a faith or a philosophy challenged by loss.

Ghandi said it quite succinctly, I believe, Spirituality is a part of you, it's something that cannot be separated from your thinking, action-taking, self. It's who you are, your morals, your values, what brings you joy.

Religion, according to the Merriam-Webster Dictionary is a personal set or institutionalized system of religious attitudes, beliefs, and practices. In other words, if you actively follow a religion, you adhere to its rules, you practice its rituals and you usually associate with other members of the same religion.

My definition of spirituality is believing in a higher power beyond myself. Religion is going to a meeting place with people of similar beliefs and go through rituals with leaders of your church. You may find comfort in the rituals that your faith community provides, including rituals offered during illness and after the death of a love one. Or you may feel the need to look deeper inside yourself, examining and perhaps even modifying your beliefs as you adjust to life without the person you loved. This may be true especially when the loss was sudden, traumatic, or intentional. As you struggle with question of spirituality after a loss, the resources of your faith can be excellent guides. Every form of spirituality, each faith, has books and teachers to turn to as you try to make sense of the loss. There also may rituals that offer comfort and assist your search for meaning. And for many, the support of a faith community can be essential.

A Letter to The American Psychiatry Association

Several years ago, you updated the Diagnostic and Statistical Manual for Mental Disorders, Fifth Edition to exclude the bereavement exclusion for the diagnosis of major depression. The public and physicians had concerns about these changes and that more people would be diagnosed with major depression. The category of grief raises the greatest concern since grief isn't a mental illness but a normal emotion of a loss that impacts every living creature's life.

The author greatest concern as a psychiatrist is that the diagnosis of Major Depression still carries a stigma in this society. Because of these changes in the DSMV it has raised fear and uncertainty that a person who suffers from normal grief will mistakenly be label with a mental illness. Therefore, the psychiatric community needs to continue to have an open conversation with the public regarding grief vs. depression. Also continued research still need to be done by the health professional community if the correct decision was made regarding the bereavement exclusion for the diagnosis of major depression and has it been validated.

Although there is some overlap in the symptoms of grief and depression they are not the same. Grief affects the heart and our emotions are colored by the shades of each individual feelings. Clinical depression affects the brain and our emotions are not colored by shades of emotions but by one emotion as if you have fallen into a dark pit, feeling hopeless, guilty and suicidal.

I have enclosed two articles that I've written to explain mental illness as a stigma in life, "The Shades of Black" that is different from a person that's grieving which can see life in different colors while they are going through the grieving process, "The Color of The Mind."

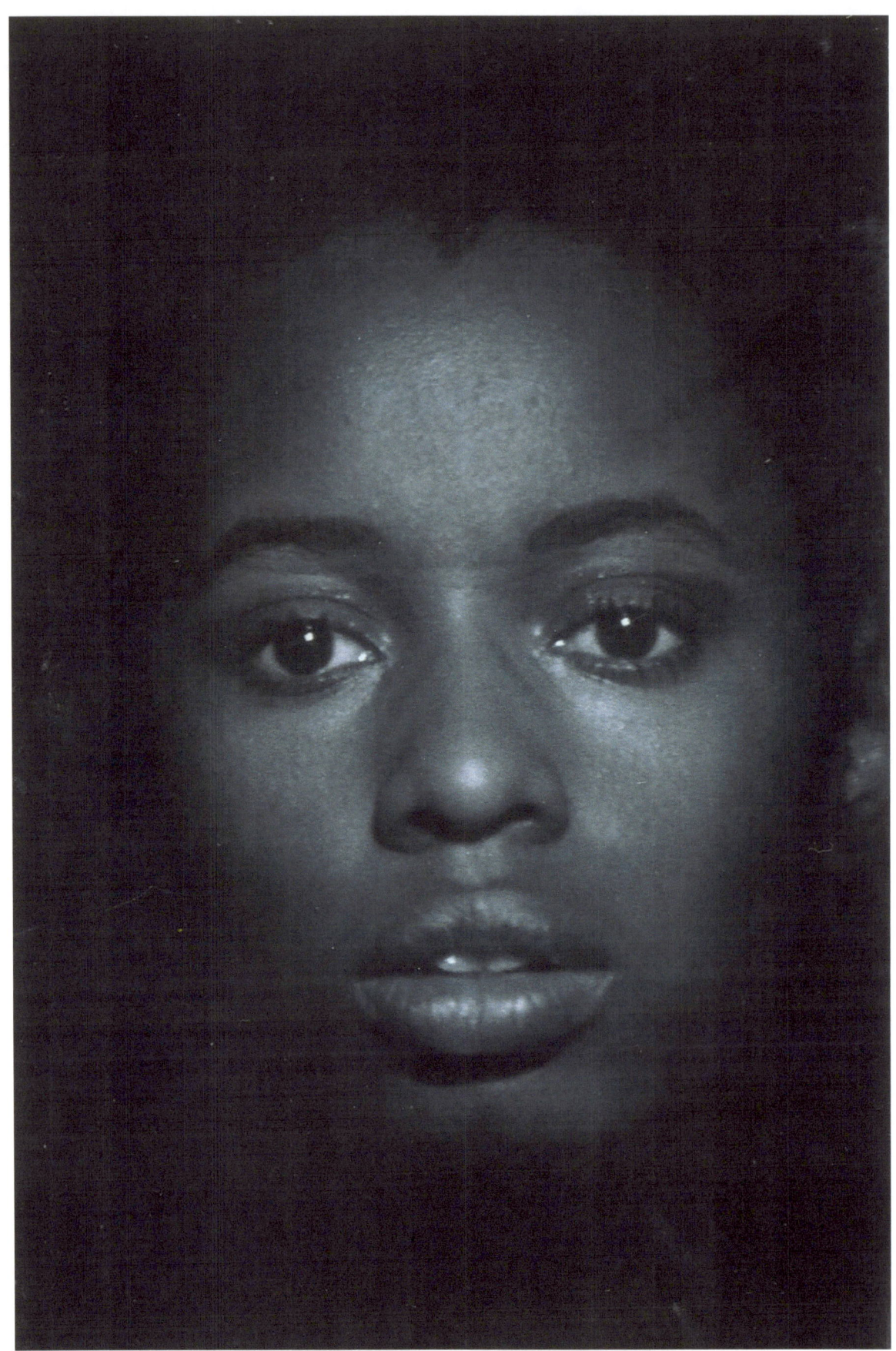

The Shades of Black

Audrey Pullman MD

Revealing the Secrets of the Brain

Seeing stars, it dreams of eternity. Hearing birds, it makes music. Smelling flowers, it is enraptured. Touching tools, it transforms the earth. But deprived of these sensory experiences, the human brain withers and dies.

Scientists long have wondered how the brain can do all the things that make one person a poet, another a builder or musician, and still another a criminal or social dropout. Until recently, medical researchers never thought they could understand the brain's inner workings. They were resigned to measuring what went into the brain and studying what came out. The brain simply considered the "black box." But now many secrets are being revealed.

Two of the most surprising and profound discoveries are that the brain uses the outside world to shape itself and that it goes through crucial periods in which brain cells must have certain kinds of stimulation to develop such powers as vision, language, smell, music control and reasoning.

Researchers have also learned that the brain patterns can be altered through brain injuries, chemical imbalance, substance abuse and genetic factors; this is also true for the body. The body is a well-balanced, biomechanically efficient structure. If that balance is altered for any reason, the body becomes mechanically disadvantaged, creating imbalances that cause structures to shift in order to compensate for the imbalance. In other words, you get sick.

The Mental Illness Stigma (*Shades of Black*)

Psychiatric disability is complex and variable in both onset of illness and long-term outcomes. There are over 57 million Americans—26% of the country—live with a diagnosable mental Illness in any given year. Yet two-thirds of those affected never seek treatment in large part due to the stigma of being labeled "mentally ill," and the resulting discrimination in social relationships, housing and employment. Mental illnesses remain the leading cause of disability in the U.S., costing society over $190 billion annually. To complicate matters, if you have both a mental and physical disabilities you have additional challenges to overcome. The many misconceptions, fears and biases people have about mental health and the stigma these attitudes create has not improve significantly over the years.

Stigma may be obvious and direct, such as someone making a negative remark about your mental health condition or your treatment. Or it can be subtle, such as someone assuming you could be violent or dangerous because you have a mental health condition. These and other forms of stigma can lead to feelings of anger, frustration, shame and low self-esteem—as well as discrimination at work, school and in other areas of your life. For someone with a mental

illness, the consequences of stigma can be devastating. Some of the harmful effects of stigma include:

- Trying to pretend nothing is wrong
- Refusal to seek treatment
- Rejection by family and friends
- Work or school problems or discrimination
- Difficulty finding housing
- Being subjected to physical violence or harassment
- Inadequate health insurance coverage of mental illnesses

Surprisingly, the disability advocates who fought for Equal Rights for the disability community have separated themselves from people with a mental illness. They have bought into the perception that people with psychiatric disabilities are untreatable and unmanageable without medications and medical supervision. The majority of disability leaders have a fear to address the needs of this community through their organizational services (e.g. employment/housing) conferences and workshops. They are also being excluded from participation in emergency preparedness planning for fear that they will decompensate due to their illness. Unfortunately, the perception about mental illness persist as a Big Black Hole that is filling up with nothing but darkness and most people are unable climb out of this blackness.

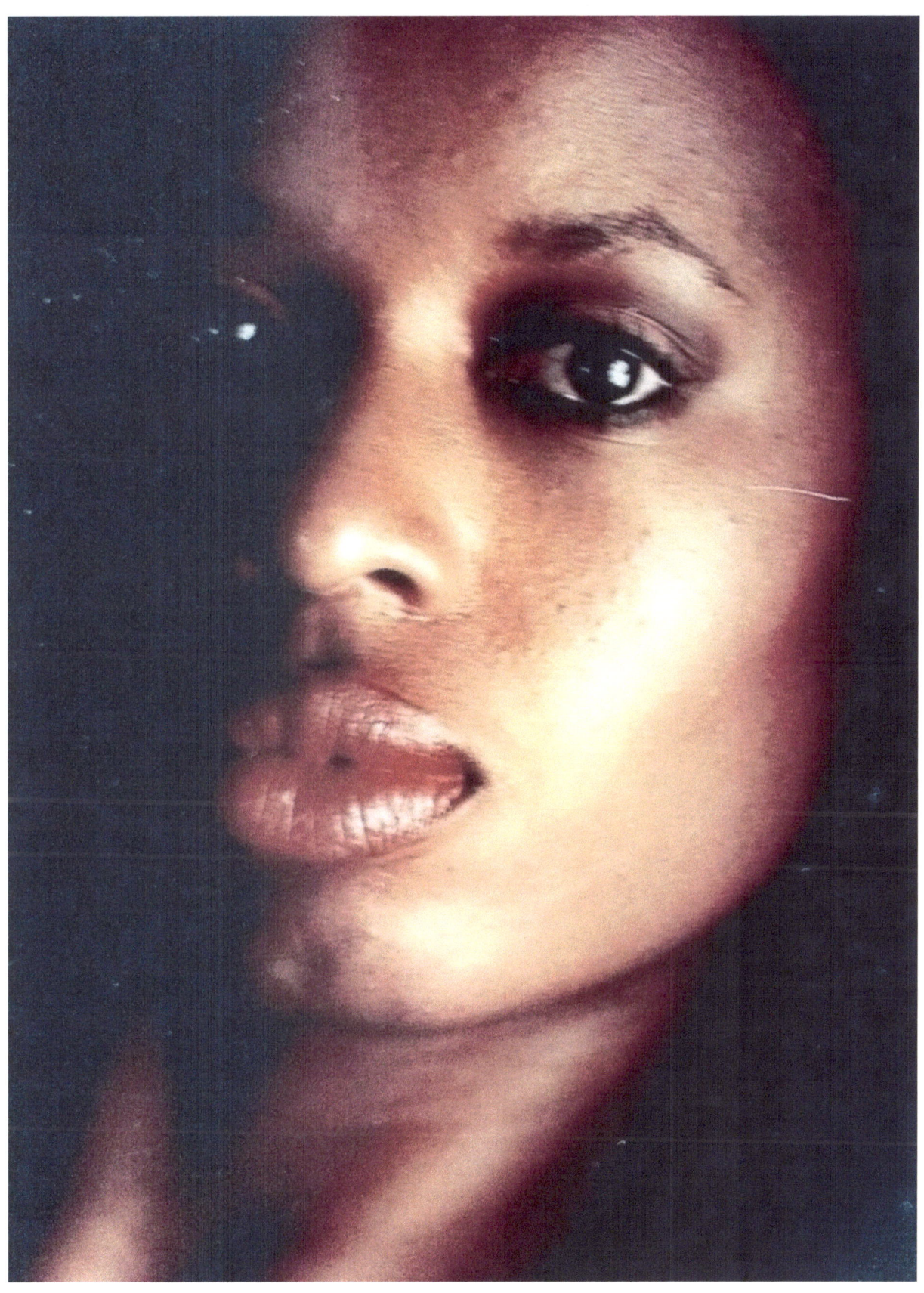

The Coloring of the Mind

Audrey Pullman, MD

Grief can be described in simple terms as shades of colors. Colors are always tough to pinpoint an emotion, simply because both are subjective and vary from person to person.

However, the Journal of Personality & Social Psychology has done studies on how color affects everything from our moods to our heart rate. Most Americans have a favorite color because color speaks a powerful, silent language. Many people associate yellow with vitality, power and feelings of positive emotions, such as their first marriage, first child and first job.

While blue is a color of clarity, communications and charm. On the downside, under stress, a "blue" person can send mixed messages, have trouble making up their mind, or just space out during conversations. Most people see red as the color of passion, anger and high blood

pressure. It is also representing the feeling of being in love (e.g. Valentine Day). The color white is light-the combinations of all colors. White symbolizes purity (the traditional bridal dress, the christening gown) and spirituality. The color Black, like white is a combination of all colors, but instead of purity, it represents the unknown, the unseen-mystery.

Black basically holds back information but there's no denying that it has strong association in our culture with "the dark side" and evil. Since color is an inseparable part of our everyday lives and its presence is evident in everything that we perceive. If people perceive psychiatric disabilities as something negative, this may evoke an emotional association with the colors grey and black; whereas a person without disabilities may evoke a positive emotion which reflects the colors yellow, blue and white. Psychologists Adams and Osgood have done a cross-cultural study of the *Affective Meaning of Color* to work with people who reflect biases and prejudice in the workplace.

Although, most psychologists view color therapy with skepticism and point out that the supposed effects of color have been exaggerated. Research has demonstrated in many cases the mood-altering effects of color have enlightened people about their biases against a class of people. The goal from the research was a self-assessment of one's own fears, anxiety, prejudice and negative emotions against another segment of population.

As a physician, I was trained that most people with mental illness will require medications along with therapy. This proved to be false with one of my therapy patients. I had received some red, white and yellow roses at my office. My client who suffered from mild depression walked into my office and noticed the roses. She marveled at the different colors, and there was an immediately positive effect on her. What happened? There was a coloring of her mind. These cool colors evoked her emotions ranging from feelings of warmth and comfort; which shifted her thoughts; which shifted her mood; which lifted her mind and spirit.

The Dialogue

This is a brief synopsis to begin a dialogue with disability advocates to gain a better understanding and openness about people with psychiatric disability. Simply remember, "that one size doesn't fit all." For example, major depression affects roughly 15 million Americans and comes in various degrees; mild, moderate and severe just like shades of colors. Given the diversity of causes (e.g. genetics, chronic stress and trauma), some people may or may not need medications.

There is a whole list of alternative treatments that people are being exposed to (e.g. creative self-expression, journaling, acupuncture & etc.) in combination of lifestyle adaptation, therapeutic techniques to communicate their darkest feelings without getting stuck in them.

Disability advocates and community leaders can strengthen their relationships through better communication and understanding with this community. Also, that people with psychiatric disabilities are a part of your community and *"want what you want."* To be treated with respect and dignity; and be a part of the planning team in every phases of emergency planning.

It is also noted that people with psychiatric disabilities issues have not been addressed at disability conferences, meetings and workshops.

Title II of the Americans with Disabilities Act (ADA) states that "no qualified person with a Disability shall be excluded from participation in or denied benefits of the services, programs or activities of a public entity" (42 U.S.C. 12131-12133, 1990). The ADA also states as a "mental impairment that substantially limits one or more of the major life activities" (U.S. Equal Employment Opportunity Commission (EEOC), 1990).

The Good News! There are a lot of support and various treatments for people who suffered from depression. The key is to find a competent physician who doesn't only has a focused-medication philosophy but who is multi-facet in his or her treatment plan

Reference List

U.S. Equal Employment Opportunity Commission (EEOC). (1990). *The Americans with Disabilities Act of 1990, Titles I and V*. Retrieved February 26, 2006, from http://www.eeoc.gov/policy/ada.html

Kotulak, Ronald (1996). The Brain, pp.1-50

Burns, David, MD (1999). The Feeling Good Handbook, pp.18-22.

BringChange2Mind.org. The Bring Change To Mind Principles, they will serve to tackle the fears and stigma of mental illness.

Israel, Toby, (2010). The Journal of Personality & Social Psychology, pp.39-41.

Adams, F. M., & Osgood, C.E (2003). A cross-cultural study of the affective meaning of color. *Journal of Cross-Cultural Psychology,7,pp.135-157.*

Conclusion – a new life path

Life isn't for the weak. Each human being has experienced good and bad times in life. Some people commit suicide because life's problems overwhelms them. The survivors of life's twist and turns must have a special place to go to find inner peace and calmness to maintain the emotional balance of living.

It's only when you develop a little understanding towards life, you will begin to try something different with your life. These are the people, who show courage to look into their lives and stand up for themselves but still, there are a few, who simply get lost in the middle of the path, and never try to see life, beyond their usual path.

People don't know, that they have the power to design their life, the way the building and car get designed. They also have the power to run their life, the way they want, and if the need arises, they can also change and modify their life.

As you grieved, look at your life, and ask yourself, do you have any control over your life? If you have control, only then you can create something fresh out of it. Only when you can consciously manage your life, you can bring the necessary changes with it. The process of life evolves in a way, where you not only manage your life but while going through the process, you understand the process of life and rise above it.

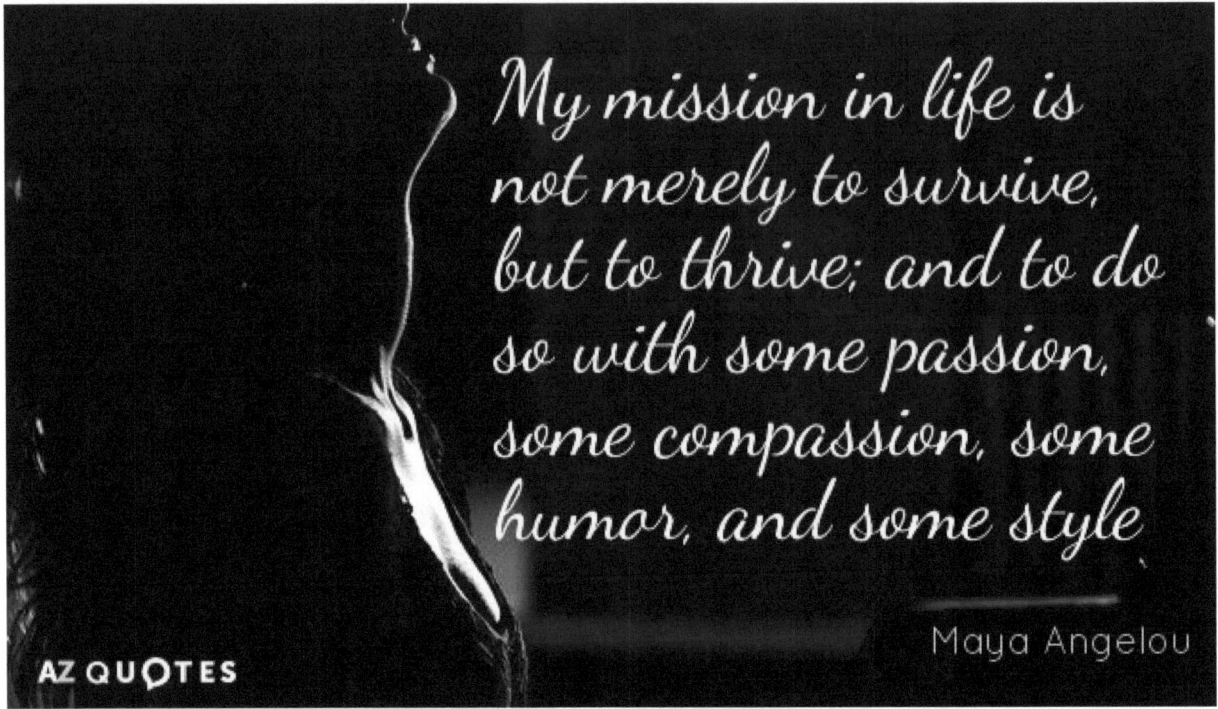